Your Diet
After Fifty

Your Diet
After Fifty

Suresh Chandra

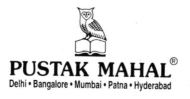

PUSTAK MAHAL®
Delhi • Bangalore • Mumbai • Patna • Hyderabad

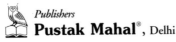

Publishers

Pustak Mahal®, Delhi

J-3/16 , Daryaganj, New Delhi-110002
☎ 23276539, 23272783, 23272784 • *Fax:* 011-23260518
E-mail: info@pustakmahal.com • *Website:* www.pustakmahal.com

Sales Centre
10-B, Netaji Subhash Marg, Daryaganj, New Delhi-110002
☎ 23268292, 23268293, 23279900 • *Fax:* 011-23280567
E-mail: rapidexdelhi@indiatimes.com

Branch Offices
Bangalore: ☎ 22234025 • *Telefax:* 22240209
E-mail: pmblr@sancharnet.in • pustak@sancharnet.in
Mumbai: ☎ 22010941
E-mail: rapidex@bom5.vsnl.net.in
Patna: ☎ 3294193 • *Telefax:* 0612-2302719
E-mail: rapidexptn@rediffmail.com
Hyderabad: *Telefax:* 040-24737290
E-mail: pustakmahalhyd@yahoo.co.in

© **Pustak Mahal, Delhi**

ISBN 978-81-223-0781-8

Edition : 2009

Printed at : Pushp Print Service, Delhi

Contents ━━━━━━━━━━━━━━━━━━━━━

Introduction **9-11**

1. **Food** **12-20**
   - Functions of Food
   - Concept of Balanced Diet
   - Planning Balanced Diet
   - Nutrition for the Aged

2. **The Concept of Health** **21-23**
   - Physical, Mental, Social and
     Spiritual Health
   - Inter-relationship between
     Nutrition and Health

3. **Nutrients: Macro and Micro** **24-52**

   a) *Macro-nutrients*
   - Carbohydrates
   - Fats
   - Proteins

   b) *Micro-nutrients*
   - Vitamins
   - Minerals

   c) *Some other elements*
   - Fibre
   - Caffeine
   - Alcoholic Beverages

- Water
- Dietary Supplements — Use and Abuse

4. The Digestive Tract **53-62**

- The Mouth
- The Swallowing Scene
- The Stomach
- The Small Intestine
- The Colon or Large Intestine
- The Appendix in the Patient Over Fifty

5. The Support Systems for Digestion **63-68**

- Gall-bladder
- The Pancreas
- The Liver Lifeline
- How to keep the system young?

6. The Principles of Eating Well **69-76**

- Supply of Energy
- Major Source of Pleasure
- Shaping Behaviour
- Health and Pleasure are not Mutually Exclusive
- Social Interaction
- Defines our Culture and Personal Identity
- Some Impediments to Eating Well
- Some Tips to Make Food Tastier

7. The Problem of Weight **77-83**

- A Longer Life
- Fasting
- A Simple Way to Reduce Weight
- Summary of Basic Facts about Weight
- Some Tips for Weight Gain

8. **Some Old age Diseases related to Food** **84-112**

- High Blood Pressure
- Diabetes
- Heart Disease
- Cancer
- Constipation
- Gas
- Haemorrhoids (Piles)
- Heartburn
- Ulcers
- Gallstones
- Osteoporosis
- Loss of Teeth
- Preventing Cavities

9. **Foods as Medicine** **113-143**

- Fruits
- Vegetables
- Pulses
- Cereals
- Milk, Curd, Honey
- Dietary recommendations for some common health concerns

10. **Fasting as a Way to prevent Old age** **144-150**

- Keep Clean Inside
- An Experiment
- Toxic Acid Crystal Theory and Back Pains
- Fasting Theory
- Subnutrition Diet

INTRODUCTION

Old adults don't fit into one neat category. Their ages span more than three decades—from their 50s into their 80s. Some live a fully active life, while others are sedentary or bed-ridden. Calendar ages have less to do with the definition and needs of ageing, however, than overall health and attitude does.

You can't stop the clock. But you can feel good longer.

Sometimes you may like to reverse the clock and wish you were 16 again, maybe 25. It is not possible to fulfil such wild dreams but you can start living a more active, healthier and enjoyable life. It is not too late to start—no matter what your age is now.

Anyone who has lived a while already knows something about staying healthy. The three key elements of remaining healthy are diet, exercise and sleep. You are doing something already in all the three directions but acquiring more knowledge and making more efforts to stay healthy should not stop. Staying fit physically, mentally and spiritually are lifelong goals.

How to eat and what to eat has a lot to do with how you age. The three guideposts—variety, balance and moderation—remain of utmost importance in the field of eating. There is a lot you can learn about nutrition and ageing. The older years differ for each individual depending on one's health and activity.

As an older adult, you need the same nutrients—protein, carbohydrate, fat, vitamins, minerals and water—as younger folks, but in differing amounts. However, a few nutrients may require special attention. Protein, calcium, vitamin D, vitamin C, iron, vitamin A, folic acid, vitamin B-12, zinc and water. Eating enough fibre-rich foods aids digestion and helps prevent the discomfort of constipation.

Energy: Spending Calories Wisely

As people get older, most use less energy or calories than they did in younger years. That is because basic body processes use energy at a slower rate and many older adults live a less active lifestyle. Yet, people need plenty of nutrients to stay healthy.

So here is a challenge for older adults. Get about the same amount of nutrients but with fewer calories. That means choosing mostly nutrient-dense foods from various food groups. These foods supply the proteins, vitamins and minerals you need for health.

Three Fundamentals of Foods:

1. Diet is important and can never be disregarded in any assessment of your health but nutrition cannot stand alone. Sometimes some other factors may interact with the food you eat or even overwhelm the significance of food. For example, in families with elevated blood cholesterol levels, drugs must supplement diet. Actually, in this case, drugs are more important than diet in lowering the cholesterol level.

2. At times too much of a good thing can cause injury. Drinking water is a very good thing but if you start taking too much of it and that also constantly, the salt content of blood may decline and you may feel weak. Chronic overdoses of water by mouth can injure kidney function, produce weakness and confusion and lead to what is known as "water intoxication." And most important, older persons are more susceptible to this threat.

   Taking vitamins is good for health but too much of them may harm your health. Nicotinic (also known as Niacin—

a member of the B-Complex vitamin family) has very good medical uses. Its large doses, perhaps as much as 2 to 6 gms. daily, are given to lower elevated cholesterol as it impairs the ability of the liver cells to make cholesterol. But too much of these doses can damage the liver and it should always be taken under close medical supervision.

3. Although there is a lot of helpful information on nutrition available these days, yet there is plenty of wrong information also. So it is important to use good judgement even as you experiment with food strategies and supplements that are the cutting edge of current research. During casual conversation people may advocate honey, garlic or some such food for treating ailments. These are useful up to an extent but your disease may be in an advanced stage and merely taking a particular food item may not do any good or may even prove to be harmful.

Also, this book is an adjunct to and not a substitute for a physician. The information contained in this book does not constitute medical advice. For any medical advice, you should consult your physician.

This book is based on the latest scientific information. Since science is always evolving, further understanding of human nutrition may lead to changes in the recommendations contained herein.

One of my goals in writing this book is to help increase your understanding of how powerful food choices can be in affecting your health and well-being. Another goal is to strengthen the communication between you and your doctor. After reading the book you can discuss your problems with him/her and both can effectively help you achieve greater health and happiness.

FOOD

The word 'food' brings to mind countless images. Food is associated with worship and divinity, with celebration and mourning, with family gatherings and feasting. It is closely interwoven with every feature of our existence. In fact, food plays a crucial role in our lives. It sustains us, it nourishes us, it is the 'life giver'.

The term food refers to anything that nourishes the body. It includes solids, semi-solids and liquids which can be consumed and help to sustain the body and keep it healthy.

Food is essential because it contains substances which perform important functions in our body. These substances are called nutrients. If these nutrients are not present in our food in sufficient quantity, the result is ill health and in some cases, even death. Food may contain certain non-nutrients as well, such as colouring and flavouring agents.

Functions:

Food has three basic physiological functions—energy-giving, body-building and protective/regulatory functions. It is also a fact that food performs these functions because of the specific nutrients it contains. Foods rich in carbohydrates or fats or both, provide energy, for instance. Similarly, foods rich in protein aid in body-building or, in other words, the addition of new tissues and repair of worn-out tissues. Vitamins and minerals present in food contribute to preventing disease. This is called the protective function. Water, fibre and, of course, vitamins and minerals play a role in regulating body functions. Food can be classified into the following three categories based on functions:

Group 1. Energy-giving foods.

Group 2. Body-building foods.

Group 3. Protective/regulatory foods.

The energy-giving category includes three types of foods:

1. Carbohydrate-rich foods A	— Cereals
	— Roots and tubers
2. Carbohydrate-rich foods B	— Sugar
	— Jaggery
3. Fat-rich foods	— Fats and oils

The body-building group includes those foods which are rich in protein. The group includes:

— Milk and milk products

— Meat and meat products

— Fish

— Eggs

— Pulses

— Nuts and oilseeds.

The primary nutrient provided by all these foods is protein. These foods provide several other nutrients as well, some of them in significant amounts. Nuts and oilseeds, for example, are excellent sources of fat in addition to protein.

The third food group is called the protective/regulatory group. The primary nutrients provided by foods in this group are vitamins and minerals.

Foods in the protective/regulatory category include:

Fruits	— Yellow and orange fruits (e.g. mango, papaya)
	— Citrus fruits (e.g. lemon, lime, orange)
	— Others (e.g. plum, banana)

This is a simple classification. However, it is useful in planning meals/diets and is the most commonly used classification. One has to ensure that each and every meal includes foods from the energy-giving, body-building and protective/regulatory groups. In this manner, the diet would supply all essential nutrients and become balanced.

After this simple way of classifying foods, let us try to understand how food groups can be used to plan meals. Take lunch as an example:

Meal: Lunch

Food Group	Food Items Selected	
	Alternative 1	Alternative 2
Energy-giving	Rice, fat	Wheat, fat, sugar, potato
Body-building	Rajmah	Green gram, milk
Protective/ regulatory	Onion, beans, tomato	Carrot, onion, tomato

Thus, two alternative lists of food items selected from each food group are mentioned. Now we must translate this into a list of dishes to be served. Such a list is called a menu. The following chart gives you an idea of how to convert these lists of food items into the magic of a menu.

Alternative	Name of dish	Ingredients used for Preparations
Alternative 1	Rice	Rice
	Rajmah curry	Rajmah, onion, tomato, fat
	Beans, vegetable (dry preparation)	Beans, onion, fat
Alternative 2	Chapatis	Wheat flour
	Dal	Green gram, onion, tomato, fat
	Carrot-potato vegetable	Carrot, potato, fat
	Sweet curd	Curd, sugar

Let us now take an example typical of the south for tiffin (a meal consumed in the afternoon after a heavy breakfast consumed mid-morning).

Food group	Foods selected	Menu (ingredients)
Energy-giving	Rice, fat, potato	Idlis (rice and urad dal)
Body-building	Urad dal, arhar or tur dal	Sambhar (arhar dal, lady's finger, potato, brinjal, fat)
Protective/ regulatory	Ladies finger, brinjal	

Concept of Balanced Diet

A balanced diet can be defined as one which contains different types of foods in such quantities and proportions that the need for calories, minerals, vitamins and other nutrients is adequately met and a small provision is made for extra nutrients to withstand short durations of leanness.

If you look at the definition carefully, you would realise that a balanced diet:

— consists of different types of food items
— meets the need for nutrients, and
— provides for periods of leanness when the diet may possibly not supply adequate amounts of all nutrients.

A balanced diet consists of different types of food items: A balanced diet includes a variety of foods. The major aim is to ensure that all nutrients are supplied. This can be achieved by first classifying food into groups—each group supplying certain specific nutrients and then selecting items from each food group to plan a balanced meal or diet. Including items from each food group ensures that all the nutrients will be supplied.

A balanced diet meets the nutrient needs: A balanced diet meets nutrient needs because of the amounts and proportions of the foods selected.

Balanced diets provide for periods of leanness: This implies that there is a 'safety margin' or a 'little extra' for those times when you do not meet your nutrient needs adequately. A normal individual consumes a variety of foods. It is possible that on a given day he may not consume foods in the amounts he requires.

15

Planning includes two ways:

— the selection of the right kind of foods; and

— the inclusion of suitable amounts of these foods so as to meet nutrient needs.

Prevention of nutritional deficiencies: If a person eats the right kind of foods in the required amounts, he or she will keep good health provided no other factors intervene. On the other hand, a poor eating pattern or eating too little or too much will result in poor health. These are both facets of malnutrition. When the diet supplies too little of one or more nutrients we suffer from a particular form of malnutrition called undernutrition. When the diet provides too much of one or more nutrients, overnutrition results.

The following chart indicates how food can be used to prevent nutrient deficiencies:

Various nutrient deficiencies	Preventive measures
1. Energy	Carbohydrate and fat-rich foods
	Carbohydrate-rich foods
	Cereals, roots, and tubers, fruits such as banana, mango. Sugars are the most concentrated forms of carbohydrates.
	Fat-rich foods
	Nuts, oilseeds, fish and meat containing high amounts of fat; vegetable oil, ghee, vanaspati, butter are the most concentrated sources.
2. Protein	Pulses, milk and milk products, eggs, meat, fish, nuts and oilseeds.
3. Vitamin A	Retinol
	Liver, egg yolk, cream, butter, ghee, milk.
	Yellow and orange vegetables, green leafy vegetables.
4. Vitamin D	Action of sunlight on skin.
	Animal foods like eggs, butter, fish liver oil.

Contd...

Various nutrient deficiencies	Preventive measures
5. Vitamin E	Vegetable oils, whole grains, deep green leafy vegetables, pulses, nuts and oilseeds.
6. Vitamin K	Dark green leafy vegetables, egg yolk, liver.
7. Vitamin B-1	Whole grain cereals, pulses, nuts, egg yolk, meat.
8. Vitamin B-2	Green leafy vegetables, milk, eggs, organ meats like liver, kidney.
9. Niacin	Cereals, pulses, milk, nuts and oilseeds, organ meats, fish.
10. Folic acid	Whole grain cereals, leafy vegetables, milk and eggs, organ meats like liver and kidney.
11. Vitamin B-12	Animal foods like eggs, organ meats.
12. Vitamin C	Citrus fruits, amla, guava, capsicum, green leafy vegetables, green chillies.
13. Calcium	Milk and milk products, some fish and sea foods, ragi, pulses, green leafy vegetables.
14. Phosphorus	Eggs, milk, poultry, fish, cereals are rich sources, present in most foods.
15. Iron	Liver, kidney, whole cereals and pulses (such as soyabean), green leafy vegetables.
16. Iodine	Sea foods, crops grown on soil rich in iodine. Iodized salt can be used instead of ordinary salt in most cases.
17. Sodium	Table salt in adequate quantities, milk, egg white, meat, poultry, fish, green leafy vegetables, some pulses.
18. Potassium	Fruits, vegetables, meat, poultry, fish, pulses, whole grain cereals.
19. Chloride	Include enough quantities of table salt.
20. Magnesium	Nuts, oilseeds, pulses, whole grains, sea foods, dark green leafy vegetables, fish, meat.

These facts lead us to the realisation that nutrients must be supplied to the body in the right amounts and proportions

17

for a person to remain healthy. If the diet lacks or is deficient in a particular nutrient, the body will also become deficient in that nutrient. When this deficiency is prolonged or sufficiently severe, the person starts showing signs of a nutritional deficiency disorder.

In addition to the above nutrients, fibre also has a valuable role to play in the prevention of diseases such as constipation and cancer of the colon. Fibre is a general term for substances which cannot be digested by the body.

Research over the past decade has indicated the beneficial role of fibre in the prevention of disease and promotion of health. Research has indicated that:

— Complex carbohydrates (e.g. starch) and fibre-containing foods are helpful in controlling blood sugar levels in diabetic patients.

— Some forms of fibre such as guar, pectin and lignin have a cholesterol-lowering action and, hence, may be of benefit in treatment of hyperlipidaemia (excess levels of lipids or fats in blood).

— Consumption of fibre-containing food is associated with lower chances of suffering from constipation.

— Eating fibre-rich foods may protect the individual against colon cancer.

— Consuming a diet rich in fibre may help induce satiety (or a feeling of fullness) and, thereby, prevent overeating. This has implications for preventing obesity (i.e. extreme overweight).

However, there is also evidence to suggest that very high fibre intakes can be harmful. Under such conditions, minerals such as calcium, zinc and magnesium are not available to the body. They appear to get bound to the fibre in the form of a complex.

Planning Balanced Diet

When planning a diet, you should remember that balanced diets are:

— individual specific

— region specific and

— income specific

A balanced diet is never generalised and suitable for all individuals. It is specific firstly to an individual of a given age and sex. In the case of adults, it is also specific to a given activity level—sedentary, moderate or heavy work. A balanced diet for a sedentary worker (e.g. typist or clerk) would differ from that of a heavy worker (e.g. construction labourer). A balanced diet for an infant would be very different from that of an adult. A diet for an adolescent girl would be different compared to one for an adolescent boy.

Secondly, balanced diets are always region specific. The particular foods available in a region can be used in planning. Using others would be impractical and unsuitable. There is no point in including a cereal like ragi in a diet meant for a North Indian because ragi is grown only in the south. A balanced diet for a particular region must reflect the characteristic meal patterns, the social and religious practices of that region. These factors are taken into consideration to ensure that the diet planned is acceptable.

Thirdly, balanced diets are income specific. Balanced diets for an individual of a given age and sex (and activity level where relevant) vary depending on income. A balanced diet would imply the use of all food groups—energy-giving, body-building and protective/regulatory—in each and every meal. However, the selection of foods and the amounts in which they are consumed would vary depending on income. As income increases, consumption of cereals reduces and consumption of milk and other animal protein foods, vegetables and fruits, fat and sugar, tend to increase.

Nutrition for the Aged

Good food and good health always go hand in hand but the nature of this friendly relationship becomes more complex the older we get. When you are young, you may skip a meal, eat anything that is put before you and in excessive quantity with few or no after effects. But after you pass age fifty, you begin to doubt whether:

— you eat too much

— you eat too fast

— your diet is a balanced one

— you should have eaten that dish last night.

Many problems may arise as a result of an unbalanced diet. But you must be careful about health problems that may arise due to many other factors as well, apart from an unbalanced diet. So you will have to consult your physician to chalk out a strategy to attack the problem on several fronts; balanced diet, medicine, exercise etc. **The balanced diet** for people over fifty is the same as for younger people. Everyday your meals should comprise foods that provide you with calories in these percentages:

1. Complex carbohydrates—such as vegetables, fruits and grain products—should constitute about 50 to 60 percent of the calories in your daily diet.

2. Protein (such as fish, egg, chicken, pulses etc.) should account for 15 to 20 percent of your daily calorie intake.

3. Fats (such as butter, ghee, whole milk) should be around less than 30% of the daily calorie requirement.

In other words:

● Choose a diet with plenty of grain products, vegetables and fruits.

● Choose a diet low in fat, salt and sugar.

● Eat a variety of foods.

● Drink alcohol, if at all, in moderation.

THE CONCEPT OF HEALTH

WHO (World Health Organisation) has proposed the following definition of health: "Health is a state of complete physical, mental and social well-being and not merely the absence of disease or infirmity."

The importance of this definition of health is that it brings out the positive aspect of health. Merely absence of disease is not health. A person may not be suffering from any disease but may not enjoy complete well-being. Sometimes we are not ill but feel tired and incapable of concentrating on our work. At such times we are not fully healthy. No person enjoys full health all the time but if one enjoys good health most of the time, we may call him healthy. Health has many dimensions: physical, mental, social and spiritual.

Physical Health

We are very familiar with this dimension of health. When we say a person is healthy we are generally referring to this aspect of health. A person is physically healthy if he carries normal weight according to his age and sex, his skin is of good colour and smooth, his digestion is normal, his eyes are bright and clear etc. Also, he is not suffering from any disease, has good power of concentration and is not irritable.

Mental Health

Mental health comprises:

— Freedom from internal conflicts.

— No consistent tendency to condemn or pity oneself.

— A good capacity to adjust to situations and people.
— Sensitivity to the emotional needs of others.
— Capacity to deal with other individuals with consideration and courtesy.
— Good control over one's own emotions without constantly giving into strong feelings of fear, jealousy, anger or guilt.

From the above description, it is clear that mental health is a more complex concept than physical health. A person may be normal in other ways but may have difficulty in understanding another person's viewpoint or may not be sensitive to the emotional needs of others. If such a problem is persistent and sufficiently serious in a person, he cannot be called mentally healthy in full measure.

There is a close relationship between mental and physical health. High blood pressure is a form of physical ill health. But it can be caused by constant stress and inability to handle difficult situations. Similarly, physical ill health can lead to mental illness. If a child suffers from polio and cannot compete with other children in games, he may develop a lifelong feeling of inferiority, self-pity and fear. It will prove a great obstacle in living a normal, healthy life for the child.

Social Health

If one recognises that he belongs to a family and is able to identify with a wider community he takes the first step towards social health. A socially healthy person relates to other people around him and fulfills his obligations to them. This type of health cannot be attained if one is physically or mentally unhealthy. Physical illness will make one irritable and depressed and he will never be able to have a healthy relationship with his family members and society in general.

Socially ill persons indulge in dacoities, thefts and even murders. Such persons are criminals but various illneses, physical and mental, also lead them to such a path.

Spiritual Health

Spiritual health is the most difficult to define. The concept of doing good and of not harming others, of believing in the basic forces of goodness and justice, of recognising the needs of others and trying to fulfill them and perhaps of believing in some supreme being are the characteristics of a spiritually healthy person. Following religious practices and customs does not make a person spiritually healthy. Spiritual health is more a matter of attitudes and a looking at situations and people. What is important is concern for others and a genuine desire to be helpful.

Inter-relationship between Food and Health

If a person takes the right kind of food and in appropriate quantity he will keep good health provided no other factors intervene. On the other hand, a poor eating pattern, eating too little or too much may result in poor health. The food eaten must not only be nutritious but must be wholesome, clean and free from harmful germs as well. The opposite of nutrition is malnutrition which refers to both undernutrition and overnutrition. Deficiency or excess of essential ingredients of food may result in impairment of health. For example, there is a general deficiency of Vitamin 'A' in our children which results in impaired eyesight and even blindness. But overeating of fats and carbohydrates also results in obesity which is itself a disease.

NUTRIENTS: MACRO AND MICRO

Nutrients can be divided into two classes: macro and micro. Macro nutrients are taken in large quantities and include fats, carbohydrates and proteins. Micro nutrients are consumed in small and sometimes minute quantities to make a balanced diet. These include vitamins and minerals. Fibre and water are also needed to maintain health and prevent diseases.

Macro Nutrients

Fats and carbohydrates are two of the three categories of macro nutrients (i.e. big foods) that our bodies need. The third is protein. The first two supply all the body's caloric or energy needs and protein provides structural elements for growth and repair of tissues.

All nutritional energy—which we measure in calories—originates as solar energy that has been captured and stored by green plants. Plants accomplish this feat through photosynthesis using the energy of light from the red and blue ends of the spectrum to bind carbon dioxide from the atmosphere and water from the earth into molecules of glucose, releasing oxygen in the process. Glucose, also called dextrose, grape sugar (in plants), and blood sugar (in animals), are the simplest carbohydrates, and the most basic food for cells of both plants and animals. It is the fuel many cells prefer to use in order to obtain energy.

Carbohydrates

The term carbohydrate refers to a large family of organic compounds essentially made of three elements—carbon, hydrogen and oxygen. Carbohydrates are widely distributed in plant foods. They are present in these foods in the form of sugar, starches and fibre. Foods rich in starch are rice, wheat, maize etc. Sugar is also a carbohydrate. Sugar is almost 100% carbohydrate while wheat contains 71% and rice 78%. Some fruits like banana and mango also contain carbohydrates.

Functions:

1. **Energy-giving function:** The chief function of carbohydrates is to furnish energy for the working of the body. One gram of carbohydrate provides approximately 4 calories. Carbohydrate foods are widely distributed in nature and are a cheaper source of energy. They usually provide 60-70 percent of the total calories in our diet.

2. **Protein-sparing action:** Though proteins can be broken down in the body to meet the energy need, this is not their chief function. An insufficient amount of carbohydrates in the diet will force the body to break down proteins for releasing energy instead of using them for the body's growth and development. Sufficient intake of carbohydrates will spare proteins from this energy-giving task.

3. **Utilisation of fats:** Some amount of carbohydrates are needed for the proper utilisation of fat in the body. Presence of carbohydrates in the diet prevents the body from breaking down too much fat for energy. This is harmful because too much fat breakdown can result in accumulation of by-products of fat metabolism. This is harmful for health.

The digestion of carbohydrates begins in the mouth itself. Saliva contains an enzyme called Amylose which is capable of breaking cooked starch into smaller units. But the time available for this process in the mouth is too short and hence the more one chews the food the more is the digestion of starch. There are no carbohydrate digesting enzymes in the stomach. The next phase of carbohydrate digestion takes place in the small intestines. Thus starch and sugar is broken into three simple units: glucose, fructose and galactose. In the body cells glucose is burnt to release energy. The extra glucose, which is not burnt, is converted into a substance called glycogen and is stored in liver and muscles and some is converted into fat and is stored in the body.

Fats: The Best Part of Food or the Worst

Throughout the world for at least three decades, people have heard that fat is bad for them and turned to low-fat and non-fat foods. Doctors, nutritionists and dieticians, all advise cutting fat intake to reduce the risk of heart disease and cancer, to lose weight and to live longer. High fat food like butter, sweets, cheese, nuts, meat etc. are now on NO lists because of their perceived ill effects on health and longevity. It is specially so for those above fifty. But their very forbidden nature increases their attractiveness for many.

But there is another school of thought which gives a quite different message about diet and health. It says that carbohydrates and not fats are the root cause of all evils, the cause of obesity, high blood pressure, heart disease, deficiency of energy, and feeling low. Low-carbohydrate diets based on this idea, some of which encourage people to eat meat, butter, cheese and cream, have become popular.

So what is it to be; a life with no butter, ghee, oil sweets, and meat, or one with no sugar, bread, potatoes, rice etc. Fat accounts for much of the flavour of food and also contributes to an all important quality of mouth feel, that sweetmeat sellers and chatwallas pay great attention to. They begin the preparation of most dishes by frying spices in ghee to release their flavours. Many of the flavour components of spices and other foods are fat-soluble and fat is the medium that conveys them to our taste buds. When we describe food we like as 'rich', we are usually responding to the 'pleasure provided by its contents of fat'.

What is Fat?

Fats, like carbohydrates, are a compound of carbon, hydrogen and oxygen. However, they differ from carbohydrates in structure and properties. The term 'fat' includes fats and oils which are greasy in feel and insoluble in water. The major constituents of all fats and oils are fatty acids and glycerol. The fatty acids are composed of a chain of carbon atoms with other elements like hydrogen and oxygen. Very often we come across the term 'saturated fats' and 'unsaturated fats'. Certain fatty acids have as many hydrogen atoms as the carbon chain can hold. They are called saturated fats. On the other hand, unsaturated fatty acids have the capacity to accommodate more hydrogen atoms. The most common distinction between the two is that saturated fats remain solid at room temperature such as ghee and butter while the unsaturated fats remain liquid at the same temperature such as groundnut and mustard oil.

The most common sources of fats are oils, ghee, butter etc. and they are almost 100% fats. Some other food stuffs also contain fats. Almond has more than 58%, mutton 13%, and fresh coconut 42% of fats. Even cereals, pulses and fruits have minute quantities of fats.

Functions:

1. **Concentrated source of energy**: Each gram of fat provides about 9 calories of energy. This is more than double the amount of energy supplied by a gram of carbohydrate or protein. Usually a small amount of fat is used to meet the energy needs of the body and the rest is stored under the skin and in the abdominal region.

2. **Safety valve:** You do not feel hungry for a long time after taking fats. This is because fats remain in the stomach longer and take more time to digest.

3. **Insulation and padding:** As already stated, layers of fat remain stored under the skin and act as an insulator and keep the body warm. A layer of fat is also present

around the vital organs of the body like kidney and heart. This serves as padding and protects them against injury.

4. **Carrier of vitamins:** Some vitamins are fat soluble and fats serve as carriers for them and aid in their absorption.

A secretion from the lever called bile helps in fat digestion by breaking fat into small droplets. These droplets are broken into glycerol and fatty acids and get transported through blood circulation. Blood carries them to cells where they are broken as energy sources or are stored under the skin.

Much of the bad reputation of fats is related to cholesterol.

Cholesterol

Actually cholesterol is a hard, waxy substance that occurs in many foods (especially meat, whole milk and egg yolk) and is also made by the liver. Cholesterol performs vital functions in the body. It serves as the starting material for the synthesis of important hormones—sex hormones like oestrogen and testosterone and adrenal hormones such as cortisone that regulate metabolism. The body derives vitamin D, necessary for utilisation of calcium and makes bile acids from cholesterol. Bile acids aid the digestion of dietary fats by breaking them down into smaller particles, and the body can rid itself of excess cholesterol by adding it to bile that is secreted into the small intestine during digestion. Cholesterol is also a component of the secretions of oil glands that protect the skin from dehydration and other sorts of environmental irritation.

Finally, cholesterol is vitally important as a modifier of the structure of cell membranes. The cell membranes are mostly composed of fat molecules.

As noted earlier, the liver makes cholesterol as a component of bile. The adrenal glands and sex glands make it to produce their hormones, and virtually all cells manufacture small amounts for their own membrane requirements. Diets high in saturated fats lead to increased production of cholesterol. But increased cholesterol production is only one part of the story of atherosclerosis (hardening of arteries). Equally important is the way this substance moves around the body. It moves through the body in protein coated droplets called lipoproteins of varying sizes and functions. Lipoproteins are transport vehicles made by the liver for conveying lipids (fat molecules) to and from cells. When tiny fat droplets from intestinal digestion of dietary fat enter the bloodstream after a meal, they are taken up by one class of lipoproteins called high density lipoproteins (HDL). HDL conveys the cholesterol to the liver. The liver sends them to other parts of the body through another class of transport vehicles called LDL or low density lipoproteins. HDL and LDL are also known as good and bad cholesterols. In fact, HDL and LDL are simply carriers or transport vehicles. High levels of LDL in the blood and low levels of HDL are correlated with blocking of arteries.

Dangers of Low Fat Diet

Usually physicians advise a low fat diet not only for heart patients but for the elderly in general. Sometimes the advice may carry its own dangers.

One outstanding danger of very low fat diets (10 to 20 percent of calories as fat) is essentially fatty acid deficiency. The danger is greater in vegetarian low fat diets, since they exclude fish and eggs and include seeds and oils.

The second danger of very low fat diets is increased cardiovascular risks due to excess consumption of carbohydrates and attendant changes in the serum lipid profile. In general, fat and carbohydrate substitute for each other in the diet; one goes lower and the other increases. Some people eating 10% of calories as fat eat 70% or even 80% of calories as carbohydrate—way too much—and develop high levels of serum triglycerides. In addition, men on these diets show decreased amounts of HDL alongwith abnormal LDL particles, which are smaller and denser, a form that may be linked to a high risk of atherosclerosis.

Palatability of food decreases sharply as fat calories drop below 20% of total calories. Maintaining a 10% fat diet is very difficult unless you hire a professional cook or are willing to give up the pleasure of eating.

Precautions to be Taken

Reduce the amount of saturated fat in the diet by curtailing consumption of butter, cream, whole milk and, especially, cheese made from whole milk. If you like dairy products, try to use low fat forms, such as low fat or skimmed milk and cheese made from part skimmed milk. Curtail intake of meat and poultry. Minimise consumption of palm and coconut oils.

— Strictly avoid all products containing partially hydrogenated oils of any kind.

— Buy all oils in smaller rather than larger quantities and use them up quickly once you open them. Protect all oils from light and heat.

— Never heat any oil to the point of smoking and never breathe the smoke of heated or burning fat—it is highly toxic.

— Do not eat deep fried foods in restaurants, especially fast food restaurants.

— If you deep fry foods at home, throw the oil out after cooking rather than saving it for reuse.

— Eat soyabean and foods made from them.

Proteins

The hunter-gatherer societies that preceded the rise of agriculture, accorded the highest status to those who brought back the most meat for the tribe. They were good candidates for tribal leadership.

Our attitudes towards protein are shaped by a variety of historical, cultural and social factors.

Protein is one of the three macro nutrients but it is special in the sense that it contains nitrogen, is made up of very complex molecules and gives organisms their biochemical identity. From the point of view of general nutrition, however, protein is neither more nor less special or desirable than fat and carbohydrate. The body needs all three macro nutrients in proper balance, and deficiencies of any of them are impediments to optimum health.

The quality of proteins in plant foods is poor and differs from one item to another. So in the Indian diet, dishes are prepared by using either a cereal-pulse combination as in dosa (rice and urad dal), dal-roti, rice-dal, or cereal-animal food combinations as in dalia (milk and broken wheat), rice-fish etc. Thus by judicious combination of food of animals and plant origin. the quality of food proteins can be improved.

In India, meat, fish, poultry cannot be taken by all, either due to their cost or religious beliefs. Milk is the only animal food which can be used both by vegetarians. and non-vegetarians. Although the protein content of milk is only 3.2%, it is of very good quality. Hence, a little of milk added to the basic Indian diet vastly enhances its quality.

Meat contains more than 20% of protein. Soyabean is the richest source having more than 40% protein whereas pulses, khoa, paneer, groundnut etc. have more than 20%.

Functions:

1. **Body building:** Proteins supply amino acids for building new body tissues and for maintenance of the body. For constant growth of human beings and also for continuous replacement of worn out body tissues, protein is a must.

2. **Proteins as regulatory and protective substances:** Enzymes play a vital role in the process of digestion of food and all enzymes are proteins in nature. Similarly hormones and antibodies which regulate body processes and protect it from illnesses are also proteins.

3. **Proteins as carriers:** Proteins work as carriers and help transport certain substances from one place to the other. Haemoglobin, the red-coloured protein containing substance, present in the blood carries oxygen from lungs to various body tissues and carbon dioxide from body tissues to lungs.

4. **Energy-giving function:** Proteins can also be broken down in the body to provide energy. But this is not the main function of protein and takes place only when the diet does not supply enough energy-giving nutrients such as carbohydrates and fats.

Deficiency and Excess of Protein

Protein needs are much lower than people imagine and the risk of protein deficiency for most of us is negligible. The early signs of protein deficiency are: hair and nails stop growing and wounds do not heal. Normal diets will fulfil all the needs of protein deficiency. Only people experimenting with strange, very restrictive diets, people subsisting on fruits and vegetables, for example, or alcoholics or very poor people living on starch are likely to become protein deficient.

Actually protein consumed in excess of the body's needs for growth becomes fuel that the body burns for energy. Protein is a relatively inefficient and dirty fuel compared to carbohydrate and fat. Protein molecules are very complex and the energy required to burn them may be more than the energy produced by them. Moreover, they have nitrogenous residue instead of producing water and carbon dioxide, the only waste products of the metabolism of fat and carbohydrate. Therefore, high protein diets in which much of the protein consumed winds up as fuel for energy production increase the work load on the liver and kidneys. Sensitive organs may also be exposed to toxic metabolic wastes.

So try to maintain protein intake between 10 and 20 percent of total calories. If you have kidney or liver problem, keep it lower. Eat a variety of whole grains, preferably less refined.

Research has discredited the idea that vegetable protein is incomplete and, therefore, less valuable than animal protein. In fact, vegetarians can survive longer and be more healthy than meat eaters.

Getting your protein from vegetables rather than animal foods has a number of advantages. Vegetable protein foods are cheaper and less perishable than meat and less likely to have toxic matter. Vegetable protein is more likely to have fibre. It is less concentrated than animal protein and can be taken in greater volume without overloading the system with it.

Micro Nutrients

Our body needs micro nutrients in much smaller amounts than macro nutrients—a few millionth of a gram in a day in the case of some vitamins and minerals. But it does not mean that they are of less importance than fats, carbohydrates and proteins. Deficiencies of some of these dietary elements will result in certain sickness and death and of others in impairment of the body's defences and below optimum functioning of many of its systems. The four classes of micro nutrients are vitamins, minerals, fibre and protective photochemicals.

Vitamins

Vitamins are an early twentieth century discovery and are now a bonanza for manufacturers and merchants of dietary supplements.

The 'Vita' part of the word 'Vitamin' means life. Vitamins are, in fact, vital and essential for life and health. They regulate metabolism, help in the growth and maintenance of our body and protect against diseases. Vitamins (like carbohydrates, fats and proteins) are organic compounds. Unlike these nutrients, however, vitamins are present in minute quantities in food. But we need not pop pills to meet the need for vitamins. By consuming the right types of foods we can meet our requirements for vitamins.

Some of the vitamins are soluble in water while others are soluble in fat. Hence, they are classified into two categories—fat soluble vitamins and water soluble vitamins.

Fat Soluble Vitamins

Vitamins A, D, E and K are known as fat soluble vitamins. These vitamins are, therefore, present in food in close association with fats. An interesting fact about fat soluble vitamins is that after being used for specific functions, the excess amount of these vitamins is stored in the body.

Vitamin A: Vitamin A or Retinol is found only in foods of animal origin. Animal foods like milk, butter, ghee, eggs, fish and liver are rich sources of Vitamin A. Liver oils of fish like helipat, cod and shark are the richest sources. However, you know that animal foods are expensive. Most Indians do not consume enough animal foods to meet the Vitamin A needs of the body. Hence, they depend on plant foods to meet their Vitamin A needs. Plant foods do not have retinol. They contain beta-carotene instead. The conversion of beta-carotene to Vitamin A or retinol is not very efficient in the body. In fact, only half of the beta-carotene absorbed is converted to retinol. Thus, people who consume less animal foods need to consume enough plant foods such as green leafy vegetables and orange-yellow fruits to meet Vitamin A needs.

Functions:

1. Helps eyes see normally in the dark by helping adjust to the lower level of light.
2. Promotes the growth and health of cells and tissues throughout the body.
3. Protects from infections by keeping the skin and tissues in mouth, stomach, intestines, and respiratory organs, genital and urinary tracts healthy.

34

4. Works as an antioxidant and reduces the risk of certain cancers and other diseases of ageing.

Deficiency: Leads to night blindness, or other eye problems, dry scaly skin, problems with reproduction and poor growth.

Excess: It is stored in the body and may lead to headache, dry scaly skin, liver damage, joint pain, vomiting and appetite loss. Normal food intake never results in excess but vitamins supplements may lead to the malady.

Vitamin D: Vitamin D is also called the 'Sunshine Vitamin'. This is because it is manufactured from a substance present in our skin on exposure to sunlight. As a result of this, we do not necessarily have to depend on dietary sources of Vitamin D. The easiest way of obtaining the vitamin is, in fact, enough exposure to sunlight.

If you don't get enough of this vitamin in your older years, you may have greater loss of bone mass and face the risk of softening of bones.

On the other hand, if you consume an excess amount, you may have kidney stones, weak muscles and excessive bleeding.

Old people should get more exposure, especially during winter, to the sun. Cheese, eggs and cereals also contain small amounts of Vitamin D.

Vitamin E: It works as an antioxidant, reducing the risk of health problems, such as heart disease, cancer and cataract that appear as you get older. It is found in vegetable oils, nuts and germinated wheat.

The latest research shows that Vitamin E retards the process of ageing. It has been found that a doze of 10 mg of this vitamin daily keeps youth intact for a long time to come. The National Institute of Nutrition of America has advised that persons above 65 should take it regularly. It is useful for patients suffering from Alzheimer's disease. For heart patients, it reduces the cholesterol level and is useful in angina pain, stroke and diabetes.

The American markets are full of anti-ageing creams, lipsticks, lotions and soaps containing Vitamin E. These are likely to hit the Indian markets soon.

Vitamin K: Among plant foods, green leafy vegetables like spinach, cabbage and lettuce are rich sources of Vitamin K. Other good sources include animal foods such as egg yolk, milk and organ meats like liver. Vitamin K is also manufactured by certain helpful bacteria which are normally present in the small intestine. Approximately half of the Vitamin K needed by us gets manufactured in the intestinal tract and the other half is obtained from animal and plant foods. Vitamin K plays an important role in clotting of blood and is, therefore, also termed as the 'antibleeding vitamin'. How does Vitamin K help in clotting of blood? It helps in the formation of a protein called prothrombin which, in turn, is essential for blood clotting.

Water-soluble vitamins: Vitamin C and vitamins of the B-Complex group are known as water-soluble vitamins owing to their solubility in water. Unlike the fat-soluble vitamins, these vitamins cannot be stored in our body in considerable amounts. The excess amount of these vitamins is instead excreted from the body in the urine.

Vitamin C is termed as the 'fresh food vitamin' because fresh fruits and vegetables are its major sources. Fresh citrus fruits (like orange, lime and lemon) and other fruits and vegetables like guava, amla, papaya, green leafy vegetables, tomatoes, green chillies and capsicum are some of the excellent sources of Vitamin C. Root vegetables like potato and sweet potato contain small amounts of the vitamin and they contribute significant amounts only when consumed in large quantities. Cereals and pulses as such are poor in Vitamin C but when sprouted and fermented, become good sources. Animal foods like fish, meat, milk, poultry and eggs contain little or no Vitamin C.

Fruits like amla, guava, green leafy vegetables and green chillies are examples of some of the cheap sources of

Vitamin C. In fact, amla is the cheapest source and provides 20 times or more ascorbic acid as compared to the expensive citrus fruits.

Functions:

— Plays a role in healing of wounds.

— Aids in the absorption of iron, a mineral which plays a role in blood formation.

— Helps overcome conditions of injury, infection and other stresses.

— Prevents destruction of certain substances present in the body as well as in some foodstuffs.

Vitamins of the B-Complex Group

As the name indicates, this is a group of vitamins with similar functions. Vitamins of the B-Complex group include thiamine (B_1), riboflavin (B_2), folic acid, niacin and Vitamin B_{12}. They usually occur together in foods. The B vitamin acts as coenzymes and helps in the metabolism of carbohydrates, proteins and fats. Coenzymes are substances which are needed by enzymes to do their job effectively. Hence, they can be considered as the helpers of 'specific enzymes'.

Thiamine or B_1: Thiamine or B_1 is widely distributed in animal and plant foods. Almost all the foodstuffs except fats, oils and sugar, contain small amounts of thiamine. Plant foods such as whole grain cereals (i.e. wheat and rice) and whole pulses are also rich sources of thiamine. Among the foods of animal origin, lean meats, poultry and egg yolk are good sources.

Riboflavin or B_2: Riboflavin or B_2 is widely distributed in plant and animal foods. Milk, liver, kidney, eggs and green leafy vegetables are good sources of riboflavin. Whole grain cereals and pulses contain fair amounts. On refining there is some loss of the vitamin. However, sprouting and fermentation of whole grain cereals and pulses can markedly increase their content of riboflavin and other B vitamins. An average mixed diet including milk, green leafy vegetables, whole cereals and pulses (especially when sprouted) can take care of the riboflavin needs of vegetarians. Non-vegetarians can also obtain riboflavin from animal foods.

Niacin: Niacin is another member of the B-Complex family. The good sources of niacin include meat, fish, poultry, cereals, pulses and oilseeds. One interesting point about niacin is that it can also be formed in the body from an amino acid called 'tryptophan'. Milk is a good example of a food rich in tryptophan but not in niacin. The tryptophan present in milk protein can be converted to niacin in the body. Thus, milk provides appreciable amounts of niacin.

Niacin (like riboflavin) is also part of coenzymes which help release energy from the end products of the digestion of carbohydrates, fats and proteins.

Folic acid: Folic acid is also widely distributed in foods. Green leafy vegetables and organ meats (like liver and kidney) are very rich sources of folic acid. Whole grain cereals, pulses, eggs and dairy products are also good sources of folic acid.

After absorption folic acid is taken to various body tissues through the bloodstream for specific functions.

Folic acid plays an important role in blood formation. You may be aware that blood has three kinds of cells—red blood cells, white blood cells and platelets—suspended in a fluid called plasma. Folic acid is important for the proper development of red blood cells.

Vitamin B_{12} or Cobalamin: Vitamin B_{12} or cobalamin is present only in foods of animal origin. Liver, kidney, milk, eggs, and sea foods (e.g. shrimps, crabs, lobsters) are rich sources of Vitamin B_{12}. Plant foods do not contain the vitamin. Vitamin B_{12} is also synthesised in our body in the intestinal tract by certain helpful bacteria.

Vitamin B_{12} can only be absorbed in the presence of a specific chemical substance called intrinsic factor. This substance is secreted by the cells of the stomach. Vitamin B_{12} is ingested and combines with intrinsic factor and is absorbed from the small intestine. Bacteria present in the intestine can also produce Vitamin B_{12}.

Simple Ways to Keep Vitamins in Food:

— Leave edible skins on vegetables and fruits or trim away as little as possible.

— Cook vegetables or fruits in as small amount of water as possible and in covered pots.

— Cut vegetables that need to be cooked longer, but in larger pieces.

— Eat vegetables and fruits raw. If use of insecticides, pesticides or ripening chemicals is suspected, then washing and cooking is necessary.

— Save liquid from cooking vegetables and add it to soups and sauces.

— Cook vegetables and pulses without adding baking soda.

— Keep milk in opaque containers. Sunlight destroys vitamins.

Minerals

The term 'minerals' may conjure up thoughts of rock. But to our body, minerals are another group of essential nutrients needed to both regulate the body process and give our body structure.

Minerals are defined as those elements which largely remain as ash when plant or animal tissues are completely burnt. Like vitamins, minerals are micro nutrients which perform regulatory and protective functions. The human body contains as many as 19 minerals in widely varying amounts. The total mineral content of the body is, however, small and accounts for only 4-6 percent of the total body weight. Some of the important minerals found in the body include calcium, phosphorous, iron, iodine, sodium, potassium, zinc and chloride. All of these minerals are, of course, derived from the food we eat.

Some minerals are required in larger amounts and others in smaller amounts.

Calcium and Phosphorus

Of all the minerals found in our body, calcium and phosphorus are by far present in the largest amount. Together these two minerals account for 75 percent of the total mineral content of the body. The human body contains approximately 1200 g of calcium, most of which is present in bones and teeth and the remaining in soft tissues and in the body-fluids. On the other hand, only 400-700 g of phosphorus is contained in the body. Like calcium most of it is also present in bones and teeth and the remaining in soft tissues and body fluids.

Functions:

Calcium and phosphorus basically serve two important functions in the body—one relating to the development of bones and teeth and the other to the regulation of body processes.

1. **Development of bones and teeth:** Calcium and phosphorus are mainly present in bones and teeth. The ratio of calcium and phosphorus in the bones is roughly 2 : 1. Calcium in the bone combines with phosphorus, some other minerals and water to form a compound. It is this compound which provides rigidity and firmness to bones. Teeth, like bones, also require calcium for their proper development. It is for this reason that the need for calcium is the most during the growing years.

   Regulation of body process: Apart from building bones and teeth, calcium and phosphorus perform regulatory functions as well. As adults get older, calcium needs go up. For both men and women over 50% calcium requirements are increased by 20%. The risk of osteoporosis goes up with age. Hip bone fractures are common among the aged and deficiency of calcium is one of the reasons. But there is one good news. If you are not consuming enough calcium, it is not too late to consume more. Consumption of enough Vitamin D and some form of exercise along with intake of calcium will prevent many fractures so common in old age.

Calcium helps in:

(a) regulating the contraction and relaxation of muscles, especially that of the heart.

(b) regulating the passage of substances into and out of the cells.

(c) conveying messages from one nerve cell to another, and

(d) the clotting of blood.

Phosphorus also performs several important functions. It is required for the:

(a) formation of a substance which aids in transport of fat in the blood.

(b) synthesis of certain coenzymes which play a crucial role in metabolism.

(c) formation of certain basic genetic material. This genetic material is involved in passing on of specific characteristics from parents to children, and

(d) capture and storage of vital energy in the cells of many tissues by forming a high energy compound. Muscle tissue is a prominent example where phosphorus helps in energy storage and thus fuels muscle contraction.

Food sources: Milk and milk products like curd, khoa, chhena (cottage cheese) are excellent sources of calcium. Foods like fish (e.g. chingri, chela) especially dried fish and other sea foods (e.g. crab, shrimp) provide substantial quantities of calcium.

Among the plant sources, ragi (a millet grown in south India) is particularly rich in calcium. Pulses like Bengal gram, green gram, moth, beans, rajmah and soyabean contribute substantial amounts of calcium. Green leafy vegetables (like amaranth leaves, colocasia leaves, fenugreek leaves, mustard leaves) also contain good amounts. Among nuts and oilseeds, gingelly (til) seed is particularly rich in calcium. Others like coconut, almonds, walnuts have a fairly good amount of calcium.

As for the sources of phosphorus, a diet that furnishes enough protein and calcium would normally provide sufficient phosphorus. Eggs, milk, poultry, fish are excellent sources of phosphorus. Cereals too are rich sources of this mineral.

Iron

Iron is a trace element present in the body to the extent of 3-5g. Most of it is found in the blood (about 75 percent). All cells and tissues, especially the muscle tissues, contain a little iron (about 5 percent) and the rest of the iron (about 20 percent) is stored in the body organs such as the liver, spleen, kidney and bone marrow collectively.

Functions:

The study of iron and its functions is fascinating. After many years of research, there are still many puzzling aspects about the role of iron especially about those related to brain functioning. Let us now study some of the known and well established functions of iron.

(a) **Oxygen transport:** Iron is a major constituent of a red-coloured compound called haemoglobin present in the blood. Haemoglobin is necessary for transport of oxygen to various parts of the body. Haemoglobin carries oxygen from the lungs to the tissues and in turn helps in carrying carbon dioxide from the tissues to the lungs. From the lungs, carbon dioxide is then exhaled. Carbon dioxide, in fact, is a waste product formed in all cells as a result of metabolism and it needs to be removed from the body.

(b) **Provision of oxygen for muscle contraction:** Iron is also present in the muscle in the form of myoglobin.

Myoglobin has the capacity to store oxygen. This oxygen is used for muscle contraction and for other immediate needs of the muscle cells.

(c) **Promotion of oxidation within cells:** Iron facilitates the complete oxidation of carbohydrates, fats and proteins within the cell. This, of course, would result in the release of the energy locked up in these molecules. The role of iron in oxygen transport and release of energy is now clear. You know that energy is required for the various physical activities we perform everyday. This is the reason why iron is crucial in helping us perform physical work.

(d) Iron plays an important role in maintenance of specific brain functions like immediate memory, capacity to learn and attention span.

(e) Iron forms a vital component of certain enzymes and substances that aid in metabolism.

(f) Iron has protective functions as well. Like Vitamin A, iron too helps in preventing infections.

Food sources: Liver is an excellent source. Other organ meats like kidney and spleen also contain substantial amounts of iron. Among the plant foods, the list of iron sources includes green leafy vegetables (like amaranth leaves, mustard leaves, colocasia leaves, mint leaves), cereals (like whole wheat flour, rice flakes, bajra, ragi, jowar) and pulses (especially the whole ones). Soyabean is an example of a pulse containing good amounts of iron. Jaggery is another food that contains fair amounts of iron.

Iodine

You would probably have noticed the packets of iodized salt. Iodized salt, in fact, is table salt to which iodine is added. The adult body contains a very small amount of iodine which amounts to only 29-30 mg. The maximum concentration of this mineral is found in the thyroid gland which is located in the neck region.

Functions:

Iodine is a component of the hormone thyroxine secreted by the thyroid gland.

Thyroxine regulates the rate of oxidation within the cell. If this regulation does not take place, both physical and mental growth will be affected. Iodine is also believed to help in the functioning of nerve and muscle tissues.

Food sources: The amount of iodine in most foods is limited and it varies widely depending on the iodine content of soil and water. Crops such as vegetables, especially those grown in coastal areas where iodine content of the soil is high, have substantial amounts of iodine. In hilly areas, however, the iodine content of both the soil and water is low. Hence, the crops grown in such areas contain little iodine.

The iodine content of animal foods like eggs, dairy products and meat depends, of course, on the iodine content of the food that is part of the animal's diet. Sea foods like fish and shell fish are among the best sources of iodine.

Another aspect that needs mentioning here is that certain plant foods like cabbage, cauliflower, raddish, ladies finger, groundnuts and oilseeds contain substances called goitrogens which interfere with the body's ability to produce and use thyroxine. Goitrogens can be easily destroyed through cooking. Hence, it is advisable to cook the foods mentioned above properly before eating.

Sodium (Salt)

Throughout recorded history, salt has played an important economic and political role. The ancient Greeks valued salt so highly that they used it for currency. Salt was even traded for slaves, hence, the phrase 'He is not worth his salt'. Roman soldiers were given a handful of salt everyday. In India, if somebody ate the salt given by the other, it made the former a loyal servant of the latter. Mahatma Gandhi started the great movement for India's freedom through Salt Satyagraha.

Although we often refer to them in one breath, salt and sodium are not the same thing. Table salt is actually the common name for sodium chloride. It is 40 percent sodium and 60 percent chloride.

Functions:

Some of the important functions of sodium are listed here:

(a) **Regulating the balance of extracellular and intracellular fluids:** Sodium, the principal mineral in extracellular fluid, is responsible for maintaining fluid balance. By fluid balance we mean the process of maintaining a balance between the fluid present within the cells (intracellular) and that circulating outside the cells (extracellular). Sodium alongwith potassium (another mineral) help maintain this balance.

(b) **Regulating the alkalinity and acidity of the body fluids:** Sodium tends to make the body fluids alkaline. Another mineral, namely chloride, present in the body fluids, tends to make them acidic. Sodium combines with chloride in the fluid and together they help in maintaining the balance of the alkalinity and acidity of body fluids.

(c) Aiding in the passage of messages from one nerve cell to another.

(d) Aiding the contraction of muscles, and

(e) Regulating the passage of substances into and out of the cells.

Food sources: You are familiar with common table salt which is nothing but sodium chloride. Common table salt is the principal source of sodium in our diet. One teaspoon of salt provides almost 2000mg. sodium. Other rich sources of sodium include milk, egg white, poultry, fish among the animal foods and green leafy vegetables (such as spinach, fenugreek leaves) and pulses among the plant sources.

Chloride

The body contains approximately 100g of chloride and most of this is found in the extracellular fluid (especially in the blood plasma). The rest of the chloride is present inside the cell. Chloride is present in the extracellular fluid as sodium chloride and in the cells as potassium chloride.

Functions:

The functions of sodium, potassium and chloride are closely interlinked. Chloride combines with sodium and potassium and helps regulate fluid balance and acidity/alkalinity of body fluids.

Food sources: Chloride is widely distributed in all plant foods. But the most important source of chloride in our diet is common table salt i.e. sodium chloride.

Potassium

Potassium is present in twice as much amount as sodium in the body. Approximately 250g of potassium is contained in the body and most of this is present in the cells i.e. in the intracellular fluid.

Functions:

(a) **Regulation of balance of intracellular and extracellular fluids:** Potassium along with sodium helps maintain fluid balance within the cell and outside the cell. As stated earlier, sodium is the main mineral present in extracellular fluid (the fluid outside the cell). Potassium, on the other hand, is the principal mineral in the intracellular fluid. Together these two minerals help maintain fluid balance.

(b) **Regulation of the alkalinity/acidity of body fluids:** Potassium, like sodium, is alkaline. It combines with chloride which is acidic and together they help maintain the acidity/alkalinity of body fluids.

(c) **Role in muscle activity:** Potassium has a significant role in the activity of skeletal and heart muscle. It helps in the transmission of messages which results in the contraction of muscle tissue.

Food sources: Potassium is widely distributed in foods. Meat, poultry and fish are good sources. Among the plant foods, pulses, fruits, vegetables, especially the green leafy vegetables, are good sources of potassium. The water of the tender coconut is, however, the best source of potassium. Among the other fruits and vegetables, bananas, potatoes, carrots, tomatoes and lemons contain appreciable amounts of this mineral. Whole grain cereals also provide some amounts of potassium.

Vitamins and Minerals

Team players: Vitamins and minerals are key to all the processes that take place in our body. But they don't work alone. Instead they work in close partnership with other nutrients to make everything happen. From helping carbohydrates, proteins and fats produce energy to assisting protein synthesis they work together.

Fibre (Our Body's Broom)

Fibre, also known as roughage, is the indigestible part of food that makes up much of the bulk of stool. Though not a source of calories, vitamins, or minerals, it contributes to health in several ways, and deficiency of it in the ordinary diet is a significant nutritional problem. Before the days of advanced milling techniques, wheat was grounded by small handmills. Such a flour contained fibre and many essential nutrients. Now a fine and white flour is a status symbol and we have lost many healthful things to it.

The easiest way to get fibre is to eat more fruits and vegetables. Psyllium seed (Isafgol) is a good source of fibre and the bulk of it makes stool larger, softer and easier to pass. It protects the health of the intestinal tract by increasing stool bulk and decreasing its transit time.

Functions:

1. Fibre prevents constipation and haemorrhoids (piles).
2. Eating plenty of fibre over the years may help prevent colon and rectal cancers.
3. Fibre-rich food may help your body keep trim.

47

4. Some types of fibres help in preventing heart disease and diabetes.

5. Taking fibre-rich food and drinking plenty of water helps reduce intestinal gas.

The Cup That Cheers—Caffeine (Tea & Coffee)

Caffeine, a mild stimulant, has been part of the human diet for centuries. As far as 5000 years ago, records suggest that the Chinese were brewing tea. About 2000 years ago, highly valued coffee beans were used in Africa as currency. Tea and coffee in the morning goes with our 'wake up' routine.

A naturally occurring substance in plants, caffeine is found in leaves and beans. We consume these products in coffee, tea and sometimes cola drinks as well. Caffeine is also used as an ingredient in many drugs and as a subtle flavouring agent.

Caffeine acts as a mild stimulant to the Central Nervous System. Some people drink tea and coffee just for that reason to keep alert and prevent fatigue.

Caffeine and Health: Over the years many studies have explored the connection between caffeine and health. No scientific evidence has been found to link moderate caffeine intake to any health risks, including cancer and cardiovascular disease.

Coffee and tea are not the best sources of fluid since caffeine can have a diuretic effect, increasing water loss through urination. The more caffeine, the greater is its potential for increasing water loss.

In varying degrees, excessive intake of caffeine may cause anxiety and insomnia. It may also increase the heart beat temporarily. In case of heart burn, peptic ulcer or acidity, hot tea or coffee may aggravate the condition.

The definition of 'excessive' caffeine intake is an individual matter depending on frequency, body weight, quantity and physical condition. If you are older, your sensitivity to caffeine may increase. At any age and specially in old age, you should pay attention to the effects that caffeine may have on you. Cut back gradually to get your body accustomed to doing with the loss. Such cutting out may result in temporary headaches or drowsiness for a few days. A gradual cut back will avoid this problem. Brewing tea for a shorter time will also help. A one-minute brew may contain just half the caffeine than a three-minute brew contains.

Alcoholic Beverages in Moderation

No one is sure who first invented beer and wine but historians do know that societies have enjoyed these beverages throughout recorded history.

In some religions, it is taboo and in India it is still not considered a good thing but we will have to concede that wine, legal or illegal, worth billions of rupees is sold every year and its sale is a good source of income for the Government.

Here I am not concerned with the religious or moral aspect of the matter. My sole concern is its effect on health and specially the health of the aged.

Although some people drink to the 'life of the party' alcohol actually is a depressant, not a stimulant. The initial 'lift' that may come with drinking is shortlived. By dulling various brain centres, alcohol may reduce concentration, coordination, and response time. It may cause drowsiness, and interfere with sleep pattern. Very often excess consumption results in slurred speech and blurred vision. It has a diuretic effect and promotes water loss.

Alcohol actually is a fermentation product of carbohydrates, both sugars and starches. It supplies energy or calories when part of food. Wine in general and beer in particular adds to body weight.

Although it supplies calories or energy, alcohol is not a nutrient. On the contrary, because alcohol may interfere with nutrient absorption, heavy drinkers may not benefit from the vitamins and minerals they consume.

For the aged, moderation is the key word. A small drink before meal may enhance appetite and add to the pleasure of eating. Consuming higher levels relates to an increased risk for high blood pressure and stroke. Excessive drinking may also lead to brain and liver damage and an inflamed pancreas.

Water

Water may also be called a macro nutrient. We require large quantities of water—more than any other nutrient to maintain our health. And water is more of a fluid to satisfy our thirst. Thirst is actually like a warning light flashing on the dash board of a car indicating that something is wrong with the engine. This physical sensation signals to you that your body needs more fluid to perform its many functions.

Water itself is a simple substance, containing just one part oxygen and two parts hydrogen. It supplies no calories. Yet every body cell, tissue, and organ and almost every life sustaining body process needs water to function. In fact, water is the nutrient your body needs in the greatest amount.

Functions:

1. Water is a major component of our body. Approximately 60% of the total body weight of an adult and 75% that of an infant is water.

2. Water is the medium of all body fluids including blood, saliva, urine, faeces, digestive juices and sweat.

3. Water plays an important role in the regulation of body temperature. The normal body temperature is maintained at 98.4°F or 37°C. Heat is produced in the body by burning carbohydrates, fats and proteins.

4. Water is a universal solvent. It dissolves a variety of substances including all the products of digestion and carries them to various parts of the body through blood.

It also helps in the removal of waste products from the body.

5. Water also acts as a lubricant by bathing the body cells and keeping them moist. It is an important part of the lubricants which are present in the joints. Water present in saliva and other digestive juices helps in the passage of food down the digestive track.

6. Water transports nutrients and oxygen to our body cells and carries waste products away. To keep our body functioning normally and to avoid dehydration, the body needs an ongoing water supply. During a strenuous workout, losing water weight is common, specially on a hot, humid day. Losing just half a kilogram of our body's water weight can trigger a feeling of thirst. With more water loss and prolonged exposure to heat, a person may suffer from heat exhaustion or risk heat stroke. A 20 percent drop in the body's water weight is defined as bare survival level.

How much is enough and when to drink: The average adult loses many glasses of water daily through perspiration, urination, bowel movements and even breathing. During hot weather or strenuous physical activity fluid loss may be much higher unlike some other nutrients. The human body does not store an extra supply of water for those times when you need more. Strenuous work, exercise, exposure to heat and even eating a high-fibre diet requires more water.

Need in old age: Thirst signals the need for water, but it is not a fool-proof mechanism, especially for elderly people. With age, the sense of thirst diminishes. So the older adults should not depend on thirst as a signal to drink water. Their kidneys may not conserve fluids as they once did. So the body holds on to less water. And those who have trouble getting around may deliberately limit the intake of water to avoid trips to the bathroom. Even in winter the evaporation from our bodies continues and we require water to replace the loss. Drinking inadequate water may lead to kidney problems and constipation. Even when you are travelling, keeping a water bottle and drinking water frequently is advisable. Here are a few tips to increase water intake:

(*i*) Drink a few sips of water even if you are not thirsty.

(*ii*) Travel with a bottle of water.

(*iii*) Drink water after 20 minutes after taking meals.

(*iv*) Milk, tea, coffee and cold drinks can be good sources of water.

Dietary Supplements—Use and Abuse

Can a vitamin or iron (mineral) pill replace dinner?

The answer is unequivocally 'no'. Food can provide the ideal mixture of vitamins, minerals and nutrients. Besides the pleasure of eating food, choices can provide the variety and balance of nutrient and other food substances needed for health—qualities that can't be duplicated with dietary supplements.

Dietary supplements include a broad range of products, whether as tablet, capsule, liquid or powder (churan). They include vitamins, minerals, fibre, and sometimes proteins as well. People take these as an easy road to health—a way that appears easier than making wise food choices. For example, Isafgol powder can be taken as a cure for constipation instead of choosing fibrous grains, vegetables and fruits.

In some conditions or after an illness, these supplements may be useful or essential on medical advice. But these should not be made a habit and necessary changes in food habits are necessary to keep good health in general. For example, iron or calcium tablets may become necessary but these cannot take the place of a regular diet containing these minerals.

THE DIGESTIVE TRACT

The Mouth

Called the oral cavity by medical professionals, the mouth is the first part of the digestive tract. This is where everything gets started and the condition of your **teeth and gums** is, therefore, the first important concern.

Digestive System

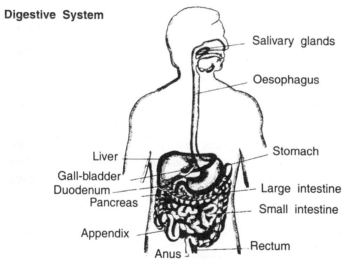

A few of the basics: Your incisors are the teeth in the very front of your mouth and are used for biting into food, the molars in the rear are intended for grinding. Good teeth play a key role in good nutrition, not to mention the enjoyment of food as the years advance. After all, if you cannot chew effectively, it limits the variety of delicious things you can eat such as the proverbial apple a day that keeps the doctor away. Pain or discomfort during chewing can discourage many old people from wanting to eat at all.

It is hard to look forward to a meal that is likely to become an ordeal rather than an occasion for satisfaction and good fellowship.

Unfortunately, a majority of people above sixty have one trouble or the other with their teeth. What causes the problems? There are two major causes. Older people have had more time to accumulate plaque, following decay in their teeth. India being a poor country with little sense of dental hygiene, some people begin to loose teeth at an early age. Proper cleaning, rinsing mouth after meals and less consumption of sugary eatables is very often neglected, which lead to early tooth decay.

In addition to cavities, old people commonly experience loosening of their teeth through gingivitis (inflammation of the gums) and other gum problems. The tendency of those over fifty to have problems with osteoporoses (loss of bone mass) may affect the bone structures in the jaw and contribute to loose teeth. The condition may lead to loosening or loss of teeth, even if he or she does not have a problem with cavities.

Tongue

Even if your teeth and gums are in a good shape, you may still find as you get older that certain foods have less appeal than they had when you were younger. Some kinds of chats, sweets and pickles may not tempt you to overeat as they did in your younger days. The reason may be the decline over the years in the sensitivity of taste buds, which have their home on your tongue.

The tongue is a mass of muscles that run in all directions. As a result of their ability to contract, the front part of the tongue can thicken, flatten, curl back on itself and move about in all parts of the mouth. It performs a double function: speech and digestion. The back of the tongue, in contrast, remains in a fixed position. The entire muscle package, that constitutes the tongue, is unique. Nowhere else in the body does a mass of muscles simply move as freely as does the tongue.

The versatility of the tongue is put to many uses. It acts as a shovel, moving food here and there under the grinding teeth. The tongue can also pass food back into the throat as the initial act of swallowing.

The surface of the healthy tongue presents an even pink-white appearance. Its lining consists of piled-up cells, comparable to those in the skin. Often, there may be a thick accumulation of cells and debris on the surface of the tongue and too much of it or unusual change in colour may occur with a fever or other health disturbances.

The accumulation of matter on the tongue is usually referred to as "fur." A furred tongue does not necessarily indicate any disease. It can be removed by a toothbrush with a light hand or with a strip of plastic or metal called a tongue-scraper.

If you look carefully at the tongue, you can see a number of little clerations all over it, resembling tiny goosebuns and other much larger mounds. It is on these clerations, which are called papillae, that a number of taste buds reside. Some, called fileform papillae, are shaped like little fingers. Others, known as fungiform papillae, look like tiny mushrooms. The most impressive of the papillae are the circumvallete type, which are located well forward the back of the tongue. Their number is eight to ten and they measure about three-eight of an inch or so in diameter.

Scattered among these cells are specialised papillae that control different nuances in the taste sensations. Scientists have identified certain groupings of taste buds that are involved in conveying sweet, sour, salty and bitter sensations. This explains why some substances can be tasted better on one part of the tongue than another. If, as a result of ageing or some other damage or deterioration, the power of a particular set of taste buds has declined, that particular food may lose its appeal or its negative impact.

The tongue undergoes quite a lot of stress and use during a lifetime, including tremendous shifts from hot to cold foods. Yet it usually withstands these assaults quite unimpaired. But some decrease in the tongue's ability to convey taste sensations can occur over time, especially for those who smoke.

Finally, a word about saliva: The taste buds respond to substances that are in solution. It is generally agreed among physicians that a perfectly dry substance cannot be tasted. Hence, the importance of the salivary glands, which pour secretions into the mouth and enhance the sense of taste.

Those who truly appreciate saliva are those deprived of it. The dry mouth feels uncomfortable; talking, swallowing, and chewing one's food become difficult. In the dry mouth, the tongue has a glazed appearance and is subject to cracks and infections. Worse yet, in the absence of saliva, teeth are highly prone to decay.

The Swallowing Scene

In a healthy state, swallowing takes place automatically and superbly and is taken for granted. But innumerable disorders may play havoc with the swallowing mechanism.

Once your food moves beyond the tongue and palate and enters the throat region, which is known as the pharynx, matters begin to get more complicated. The pharynx, as a space common to both the respiratory and digestive systems, is the scene of many air-food "traffic" problems. The food you eat must move through this area towards the stomach; the air you breathe also must be channelled through this space. All this activity makes for a lot of stop-and-go signals for the pharynx.

During most of the day, the oesophagus, or food pipe, is closed down, and the trachea, or windpipe, remains open to allow you to breathe freely. Unconsciously and automatically, your diaphragm, the muscular wall that separates your chest and abdominal cavities, descends and causes your lungs to expand. This motion pulls air into your body, generally through your nose. The air then passes down through the pharynx, into the trachea (windpipe), and finally into your lungs. When the diaphragm moves back up and presses against your lungs, you exhale through your nose to complete the breathing cycle.

But this natural process of breathing is interrupted when you take food into your body and begin to swallow. To make swallowing a success, it is necessary for your body to manage two lines of traffic: (1) air must come in from the back of the nose and be channelled down into the windpipe; and (2) food must be directed from the mouth down into the foodpipe. Obviously, there is plenty of opportunity for collisions here.

The solution to this traffic problem has been the creation of a barrier in the pharynx, so that what we eat has the "right of way." Only one route, the one that food takes through the foodpipe, has priority during a snack or meal. Our swallowing in effect shuts off the two incoming routes: No more air can be inhaled. Swallowing also erects a "stop sign" in front of the outgoing route that exhaling air takes through the windpipe.

With three of the four avenues into the pharynx thus cut off, the contraction of the muscles in that area during swallowing can, without obstruction, push the food into the only open channel, the foodpipe and finally down into the stomach.

Sometimes, however, this tidy process of traffic control goes awry, especially in older people. The muscles that produce good swallowing may decline somewhat in power and coordination with age, and as a result, there may be more of a danger of choking on food.

When such choking occurs, a piece of food typically gets caught in the trachea before it closes down during swallowing. As a result, the victim's breathing apparatus is plugged up, and if steps to dislodge the food are not taken quickly, the person may suffocate.

The highway of the oesophagus (food pipe): After your food makes it through the pharynx, the oesophagus, a ten-inch muscular tube less than a garden hose in diameter, takes over as a conduit or "highway" to the stomach. The muscles of the oesophagus propel the food along with a moderate thrust, sufficiently strong that many healthy people can swallow while in an upside-down position.

But the transit through this anatomical highway is not as rapid, or in some cases in older people, as easy as many imagine. It takes on the order of eight to ten seconds for food to traverse the ten-inch length of the oesophagus. In contrast, the musculature of a dog's oesophagus contracts much more rapidly, so that a dog can "wolf" its food down with such impressive speed.

The oesophagus has relatively few glands, and no digestion occurs in it. As a structure of the neck and chest only, it penetrates the diaphragm through an opening called the hiatus. Once through this aperture, the oesophagus enters the abdomen and there ends in the expanded portion of the digestive tract we know as the stomach.

In old age food takes longer to make its way down the food pipe because of a decrease in the wave-like motion that pushes the food towards the stomach. But this has no significant effect on digestion.

The Stomach

The centre of digestion, the stomach is the familiar receptacle at the end of the oesophagus. It is roughly the size and shape of a somewhat small, lopsided football, into which large amounts of food can be deposited. The shape of the stomach may vary considerably, depending on the person's build. In slender people, the stomach tends to be elongated and may even dip down as far as the upper part of the pelvis. On the other hand, in some short stocky individuals the stomach may have an almost sideways traverse position.

The curved upper part of the stomach known as the fundus, rises above the level at which the oesophagus enters the stomach. This upper section of the stomach rests against the diaphragm and is the place where swallowed air accumulates. It is this air that we attend to release when we belch after a meal.

Changes in old age: In the stomach production of gastric juice declines as we grow old. In the middle years, there is an increased incidence of chronic inflammation of the stomach with degeneration of mucous lining. Either or both of these changes can prevent an older body from absorbing as much iron and vitamin B_{12} as a younger one. But an improved nutrition can take over the slack.

The Small Intestine

The small intestine is composed of that portion of the digestive tract which is between the opening at the end of the stomach and the large intestine, or colon. We call this the "small" intestine because of its width, not its length.

The small intestine is about the same size in diameter as the foodpipe, but that is the only way it is small. This part of the digestive tract is at least a dozen feet in length, and it is the major organ for absorption of food and nutrients, as well as for continued digestion. Into it are poured the secretions of the pancreas and the bile secreted by the liver. All these enter on top of the digestive secretions of the intestinal cells themselves. Even in the absence of the stomach, digestion should be complete because of small intestinal activity. This is a prime example of nature's backup planning.

The first portion of the small intestine, the ten-inch duodenum is fixed in position. The C-shaped curve of the duodenum, which is sometimes referred to as the "duodenal sweep", encloses the head of the pancreas. The pancreas is the organ that secretes enzymes into the intestines for the digestion of food and also manufactures insulin, which is secreted into the bloodstream for the control of blood sugar.

In contrast to the duodenum, the rest of the small intestine is capable of some mobility. This mobility is possible because the small intestine is suspended in a loose covering membrane known as the mesentery.

The Colon or Large Intestine

The colon is readily distinguished from the small intestine because of its large size. In some ways, the large intestine bears the same relationship to the small one as a warehouse does to the factory it serves. The colon warehouse is large but performs no digestive business, other than storage. The single most important function of the colon is the absorption of fluids. Incoming wastes are gradually made more solid as fluids are absorbed into the body during the journey through the large intestine.

The bulk of the material the colon deals with involves the indigestible residues from our food. In the ordinary mixed diet, these include mostly the cellulose remnants of the vegetables and fruits we eat. A good deal of cellular debris can also be found in the stool: cast-off lining cells, various kinds of white blood cells and variable amounts of mucous secretions. These products help determine the constituency, including the hardness or softness of the stool.

On the other hand, the colour of the stool depends on the bile that enters from the liver. Slight modifications in the chemical structure of the bile pigments produce colours ranging from green to yellow, and on to brown of various shades. All of these colours are perfectly normal. They are derived from the bile, which is initially green but then is chemically altered to other shades.

The course of the colon: The colon makes two fairly sharp changes in its course through the body, a pattern that can be useful in trying to determine where some discomforts arise. The ascending colon, the first part of this organ, arises in the right lower position of the abdomen and runs in a more or less straight path upward to the liver. At this point, the colon executes a sharp turn to the left known as the hepatic flexure.

The next portion of the colon runs more or less straight across the abdomen from right to left, but may drop downward through part of its course. This is called the traverse colon. In the upper left portion of the abdomen, the organ then executes another turn known as the splenic flexure (after the spleen).

Then the colon runs more or less straight down the left side of the abdomen as the descending colon. Finally, it enters the upper portion of the pelvis, where it is sometimes referred to as the pelvic colon.

The first portion of the pelvic colon forms a configuration that has been compared to the Greek letter S or Sigma. It is, therefore, sometimes called the 'Sigmoid colon'. Below the sigmoid is a relatively straight portion of the organ that we commonly call the rectum. (Rectum is the Latin word for 'straight'.) The rectum finally emerges at the anal opening, which is the end of the digestive system.

The much longer, though narrower, small intestine enters the colon through a valve-like slit called the ilcocolic valve. Just below this entrance is a pouch-like area in the colon called the caecum, the home of one of the most famous of all abdominal organs, the appendix.

The Appendix in the Patient Over Fifty

The appendix, a three-to-five-inch pencil-size projection from the caecum, performs no digestive functions. But it can certainly create big problems in older people.

Fortunately, the appendix is a relatively uncommon cause of difficulties in elderly people. In fact, appendicitis in all age brackets seems to be on a definite decline. But appendicitis in a patient over sixty years of age does account for 6 to 8 percent of all appendectomies. So it is important to know something about this structure and about the symptoms that may arise when appendicitis strikes.

It is especially important to act quickly with a possible appendix problem as you get older. If you delay seeking medical care, there is a greater likelihood that you as a person over fifty will suffer a ruptured appendix than will those who are younger. Mortality rates among older people with a ruptured appendix can range from 7 to 9 percent.

In consideration of abdominal pain at any age, always think of acute appendicitis. Never take a laxative for abdominal pains. That may hasten a rupture.

THE SUPPORT SYSTEMS FOR DIGESTION

Gall-bladder

The gall-bladder is a hollow, pear-like structure, situated under the liver in the upper right part of the abdomen. Its function is to store and concentrate bile from the liver. The chief work of bile is to render fats more soluble, much as a detergent dissolves grease. The bile from the gall-bladder pours through a duct into the duodenum, the upper part of the small intestine.

What can go wrong with the gall-bladder: Gall-bladder disease is the most common reason for abdominal surgery in those over sixty. Specifically, there is a progressive increase in the appearance of gallstones after about age twenty, so that 25 percent of those aged around fifty to sixty have the problem; 40 percent aged around sixty to seventy have it; and the incidence rises steadily the older we get.

The most common problem presented by the gall-bladder is that of stones. Perhaps this is related to the fact that one of the chief contributions the gall-bladder makes is to concentrate the bile, which flows out of the liver. The gall-bladder stores bile and makes it into a denser fluid. Then, when a fatty meal is passed on by the stomach into the small intestine, the gall-bladder contracts and pours the concentrated bile out and over the food.

This is a sensible arrangement, with one drawback. The gall-bladder bile is so concentrated that its ability to hold its constituents in solution is limited. A trace of a foreign

63

substance, perhaps a clump of bacteria or other tissue, may become a focus for deposits of bile components, and this is the beginning of a stone.

As we know from serial X-rays, tiny gallstones tend to grow slowly larger by ongoing deposits. Their constitution also varies. Some, it turns out, are virtually pure cholesterol. Others are chiefly the bile pigment; still others are a mix of chemicals, may include calcium, and are sometimes quite large.

Stones may thus vary from tiny—under a millimetre—to grape size. Also, they are in varying shapes, including round and square. Some gall-bladders contain hundreds of small stones and others, a few grape-size ones.

What creates the problem is that the gallstones may move out from the gall-bladder, a journey that creates pain and sometimes havoc. For example, a stone may be jammed into the cystic duct. This is the small canal that leads from the gall-bladder to the main bile duct, which then runs on the intestine. The stone obstructs the channel through which gall-bladder bile is passed out creating a painful condition.

The Pancreas

Almost no one outside the medical profession seems to know what the pancreas does, except those who have a problem with this important organ.

The pancreas is a pink-white, tube-shaped organ whose appearance is somewhat like that of a salivary gland, so much so that doctors sometimes refer to it as the "abdominal salivary gland."

Plastered up against the back wall of the abdomen, this structure measures six inches in length and is divided into three portions: the head, the body and the tail. The head of the pancreas nestles within the C-shaped loop formed by the duodenum (the upper part of the small intestine). The body of the pancreas comprises the main mass of the organ; the tail is that portion that is quite close to the spleen, a lymph organ that disposes of used red blood cells.

Most of the pancreas consists of cells that secrete digestive juices that are poured out through a major duct connected to the bile duct. The pancreas is much like the salivary glands in the mouth in that pancreatic secretion contains an enzyme capable of breaking down starchy materials. In addition, this organ contains other potent enzymes capable of breaking down proteins (this enzyme is known as trypsin) and fat (the enzyme pancreatic lipase).

The Liver Lifeline

The liver far and away outperforms all other organs in the body, in terms of its total number of basic tasks. It is also the largest organ in the body, representing about 2 percent of our body weight. After we pass age fifty, the weight of the liver slowly begins to decrease. Despite this weight loss, though, we can usually depend on the liver to operate efficiently throughout our entire life, so long as we refrain from abusing it.

The place of liver and its functions: Most of the liver can be found in a space hollowed out at the arch of the diaphragm and the lower loop of the ribs. Although most of the liver is in the right upper portion of the abdomen, a large part does extend past the midline of the body and well towards the left side.

— The liver helps detoxify ammonia and various other potential toxins formed in the large intestines during digestion.

— It inactivates the female hormone oestrogen, thus setting an upper limit on the amount of this substance that circulates in the body.

Note: Small amounts of the female hormone are also produced in the male body and are deactivated by the liver. So if a man starts to show feminine characteristics such as enlargement of breasts or loss of body hair, as occasional patients have, these characteristics may indicate the presence of liver disease.

— The liver stores sugar and regulates sugar levels in the blood.

— It produces substances necessary for clotting of blood.

— It produces many of the proteins found in the bloodstream.

— It produces, stores and regulates many of the bodily fats and lipids, including the all-important cholesterol and its various subcomponents such as high-density lipoprotein (HDL) and low-density lipoprotein (LDL). HDL protects against cardiovascular disease, whereas LDL promotes it.

— It produces or stores many important vitamins, ranging from vitamins A and D to K and B_{12}.

— It sets up important defences against bacteria.

With all of the things the liver has to confront, it is not surprising that it may become inflamed, a condition known as hepatitis. This can be caused by a variety of drugs, chemicals or alcohol. Perhaps the most common cause of hepatitis, however, is viral inflammation, hence, the term viral hepatitis.

A number of viruses are capable of causing severe inflammation of the liver. The most common, dubbed hepatitis A, is spread mostly via contaminated foods. It can occur in epidemics.

Because this virus is excreted in the stool, it can be recycled through contaminated water.

It is important to know that many of us have protective antibodies, even though we may have no history of the disease. The reason is that viral hepatitis can be a silent infection and may not produce jaundice. Often, its onslaught is attributed to a "flu bug" or a "stomach upset". It has been estimated that for every case in which the diagnosis is made—usually because the person turns yellow—there are ten cases or more in which the full-fledged disease does not come forth. But protective antibodies are formed even in the mild or inapparent cases.

The liver goes through a number of age-related changes including reduction of enzyme concentrations. But this organ has a startlingly large reserve capacity. Scientists say that 80 percent of the liver can be removed without impairing its function.

How to Keep Your System Young?

The digestive tract ages. But the system itself is designed to take ageing in its stride. Here's how to keep the digestive tract functioning well for a lifetime.

— Eat a high-fibre diet; sufficient bulk in the colon keeps the system working smoothly. Lack of dietary fibre is linked to constipation and other bowel problems. High-fibre foods include: bran, whole grain, breads and cereals, fresh fruits and vegetables.

— Eliminate foods that cause you digestive distress. Some people may have problems with gas-producing vegetables like cauliflower and cabbage. Others may find milk products less and less digestible. If you suffer cramps, gas, diarrhoea or constipation, think back to what you ate during the past 48 hrs.

— Moderate calories. Overeating can cause stomach bloat, heartburn and bowel distress. High-calorie diets have been linked to gallstones.

— Practice good eating habits. Make mealtime relaxing. Don't eat on the run, eat while talking or gulp hot liquids. Following these commonsense habits can save you from indigestion, heartburn and even ulcers.

— Reduce or eliminate alcohol, caffeine and nicotine. These common and commonly abused drugs are stomach and bowel irritants and may lead to heartburn and indigestion.

— Be an aware drug consumer. Some medications are not suitable to the digestive tract. Aspirin, diuretics, antihypertensives, sedatives and other substances can cause distress. Ask your doctor about potential side effects of all medications.

— Don't overuse laxatives, antacids or other over-the-counter remedies. At best, they relieve only symptoms. At worst, they encourage the digestive tract to become dependent on something other than its own processes.

— Reduce daily stress or develop ways of coping with it. Burying tension and internalising anger are two good ways to wreak havoc on the digestive system.

— Exercise regularly. It helps control weight, reduce stress and keep the bowel functioning normally.

THE PRINCIPLES OF EATING WELL

When I use the word "eating well", I mean using food not only to influence health and well-being but to satisfy the senses providing pleasure and comfort. In addition to supplying the basic needs of the body for calories and nutrients, an optimum diet should also reduce risks of disease and fortify the body's defences and intrinsic mechanism of healing. I believe that how and what we eat is an important determinant of how we feel and how we age. I also believe that food can function as medicine to influence a variety of common ailments.

Among other things, the purpose of this book is to explore the issues and controversies surrounding food and nutrition in order to bring clarity to the subject and establish for readers, especially those over 50, a sense of what eating well means. So I want to state five basic propositions that underlie the philosophy of food and nutrition and how they influence health.

Supply of Energy

The body requires energy for all of its functions, from beating of the heart and elimination of wastes to the transmission of electrical and chemical signals in the nervous system. It gets its energy from food, by taking it in, digesting it and metabolising its components. Food is fuel that contains energy from the sun, originally captured and stored by green plants, then passed along to fruits, seeds and animals. Humans eat these foods, and burn the fuel they contain, that is, combine it with oxygen in a controlled fashion to release and capture the stored solar energy. As long as we live, we have to eat.

Not having enough food is seen as an ultimate misfortune and a cause of human suffering, and having it in abundance is a cause for rejoicing. So we must not only eat to live, whether a child, young man or elderly, but eat often.

Eating is a Major Source of Pleasure

Among the people where food is scarce, it is seen primarily as a necessity of life and little thought is given to it beyond that. But where food is abundant, people use it for purposes far beyond mere survival. Even in a poor country like India, a great deal of time, energy and money go into the preparation and consumption of food that is intended to provide pleasure. Think of the comforts foods give when you are sick, tired or sad. Remember the times during sickness when your caring parents brought you many kinds of foods which were tasty but not harmful.

Shaping Behaviour

Psychologists describe food as a primary reinforcer, that is, something with intrinsic power to shape behaviour. Food is used by trainers to elicit performances of animals in circuses and movies in apparent contrast to their wild natures. When hungry, even human beings would do almost anything to get it.

Of course, not all of us respond to food in the same way. Individuals derive various degrees of pleasure from it. For some, eating is mostly a necessity of life, attention paid to the sensual aspect of food is minimal and pleasure is sought elsewhere in music, literature etc. But still the fact remains that food is an important source of pleasure for most of us.

Health and Pleasure are not Mutually Exclusive

Some chronic patients of heart disease, diabetes and hypertension complain that their doctors have prohibited salt, sugar and fats. They are at a loss to know what they should eat. Everything they like to eat is bad for them. "Is healthy food always dull?" Of course, the food prescribed for those who suffer from a particular disease must exclude certain items which are palatable to most of us. But things can be made better if the prescribed foods are cooked and served in different ways. They need not include salt, sugar and fats.

Moreover, the quantity of so-called unhealthy food can be reduced. Attempts should be made to embrace both the aspects of foods—health promoting and pleasure giving.

Social Interaction

Coming together to share food is a behavioural pattern we have in common with many other creatures. Breaking bread together both establishes and symbolises a fundamental social bond. Think of the communal eating on the occasion of marriages, birthdays and sometimes even on the death of an elderly person. Festivals are the right occasions for feasts. *Langars* in gurudwaras and *bhandaras* on festivals are a common sight. In fact, the words *festive, festival* and *feast* have a common Latin root suggesting the occasion for merry-making, enjoying and eating in company.

The social importance of food and eating, like their association with pleasure, must be honoured. Even old people following rigid diet regimens should not isolate themselves. Social interaction in itself is an important factor in optimum health. Camaradarie is the best diet when food is blessed by being shared, by being eaten in fellowship between conversation and laughter—all such food is 'health' food.

Defines Our Cultural and Personal Identity

Special foods prepared on some festivals or occasions help identify a particular community living in a region. In Northern India, sweets of some special kinds, snacks and fried food are made on the occasions of Diwali and Holi. Similarly, Bihu in Assam and Pongal in Southern India are occasions to prepare particular types of food which are relished in those parts. Internationally, Japanese prepare Mochi on New Year's day. It is made from sticky sweet rice, traditionally and laboriously prepared in company by soaking, steaming and pounding in huge mortars with huge clubs.

Sometimes, disliked and prohibited foods have much to do with one's identity and culture. Orthodox Jews and Mohammedans will never eat pork. Similarly, for Hindus, beef is taboo. Jains are very choosy in this matter and will not take onions, garlic and sometimes even curds. Some of them eat nothing after sunset, perhaps an old tradition when there was no electricity and lighting lamps attracted insects, which might have mixed with food and contaminated it.

Often, it is culture-specific tastes and odours which people long for when they leave their native lands and settle or travel through foreign lands. The French pine for their excellent bread, Indians for curries and Japanese for their rice. Sometimes, a particular food item may be harmful to health but people stick to them. For Indians, *desi* ghee with its distinctive flavour is very appealing. It was a healthy and nutrient diet when people undertook hard physical labour but has now become the bane of life for many. It is pure butter fat, the most saturated of dietary fats and is a major contributor to atherosclerosis and coronary heart disease, which is spreading quite rapidly in India.

Eating well means, among other things, not rejecting or giving up the food that defines our personality, society or culture. Rather it means to adopt them to confirm to dietary principles that promote optimum health.

Eating is One of the Health Determinants

Just as the quality of fuel influences the performance and longevity of an internal combustion engine, so the quality of food we eat must influence the life and health of the body. The question is how great that influence is relative to other factors. Actually the determinants of health are myriad. Starting with genetics and including a great many environmental, psycho-social and spiritual factors, diet is only one aspect of lifestyle and lifestyle is only one set of variables in the mix. It is probably not possible to isolate from this complexity any one element and specify its exact contribution to health and happiness. It is a false claim that diet is the sole determinant of health or as the cliche goes: *we are what we eat.*

Nevertheless it is possible to get an idea of the influence of diet by looking at the effects of dietary changes in large populations and the increasing incidence and frequency of certain diseases. Take the case of India; we are in for a rapid dietary and lifestyle change under western influence. Increased consumption of fast food, and dairy products, combined with rising affluence and mechanisation are taking their toll. India is in for increasing numbers of coronary heart disease, diabetes and cancer as well. This lifestyle has influenced even Japan and China. The whole of South-east Asia is undergoing a change for the worse—for the time being at least. Diet has special significance among lifestyle factors in that people have total control over it, at least potentially. You cannot change your genes, control the quality of the air you breathe all the time, or avoid the stresses of everyday life, but you can decide what to eat and what not to eat even if you are stuck in a marriage feast or a birthday party. It is a shame not to take advantage of that control by making wise choices from what is available and by informing yourself about wise and unwise choices of food.

Some Impediments to Eating Well:

Chewing Problem

For many older adults, poor appetite is not much of a nutrition problem. Instead, tooth loss or mouth pain is. Tooth loss usually begins at 50 and many people lose most teeth by the age of 70. Poor fitting dentures also cause chewing problems and mouth sores.

Having a dry mouth is another problem that may cause chewing and swallowing difficulties, especially if the food is dry and hard to chew. As people get older, they may not have much saliva flow to help soften food and wash it down. Some medicines may also produce dry mouth.

If you have these problems, make sure these do not become a barrier to good nutrition.

- **Take a visit to the dentist:** An ill-fitting denture, painful tooth or soft gums can be treated easily after a few visits to the dentist.

- **Choose softer foods that are easier to chew:** Chop foods well to avoid the risk of choking. Cooked rice, dalia, soft bread, vegetables with soup, *khichdi* are some of the soft foods.

- Vegetables should be cut into small pieces and cooked well to make chewing easy.

- Fruits should be peeled and cut into small pieces. I have seen some old people making a paste of apple, guava etc. to make chewing easy.

- Intake of milk, curd, paneer etc. can be increased.

- Drink some water with food to make swallowing easy.

Loss of Appetite—Causes

There are a number of factors, which may be responsible for loss of appetite during ageing.

1. The papillae of the tongue—the small projections that contain the taste buds—often shrink with age. It results in a declining ability to distinguish among various sweet, salty, or sharp tastes. The decline in the taste buds may be due to a natural deterioration of the elements of nervous system or lower intake of Vitamin C.

2. Appetite may also decline as the sense of smell deteriorates with age. The ability to distinguish the odours of food accounts for 80 percent of flavour sensations.

3. Tooth and gum problems increase with age and these difficulties can lessen the enjoyment of food. For some people it is painful and unpleasant to chew with teeth or gum that are giving trouble. Others have dentures that may not fit quite right and thus may make it hard to chew.

4. A decrease in the efficiency of the secretions and organs in the ageing body may cause a loss of appetite. For example, the inability of the ageing stomach to produce the usual level of acid in the digestive process may cause discomfort—such as gas, cramps or simply a heavy feeling. Sometimes, the declining levels of the lactose enzyme with age may result in lactose intolerance. This may lead to gas, cramps and even diarrhoea after consumption of milk or other dairy products. Sometimes, a person living all alone may lack the self-imposed discipline of having another person for whom they have to prepare meals. This is more true for women, who—when left alone—may not cook meals both the times and consume stale or unbalanced food due to sheer laziness and indifference.

5. Inactivity may contribute to a loss of appetite. A number of studies have shown that older people increasingly take in fewer calories than their younger counterparts. It has been estimated that for each decade after age twenty-five, the number of calories the average person requires to maintain a given weight, drops by at least 2 percent. This means that by age 65, you need 8 percent fewer calories, than you did at the age of twenty-five.

Coping with this loss of appetite is possible and also necessary. Here are some tips:

— *Eat by the clock than by hunger:* Eat something at the appointed time.

— *Add some delicacies to your food:* Colourful foods, appealing texture and an appetising aroma are helpful aids to increase food intake.

— *Eat meals with friends:* The pleasure of being with others may be an appetite booster.

— *Keep favourite foods on hand—for meals and breakfast:* You may eat more when food is available.

— *Make meal times pleasant:* A relaxed and attractive setting with soft music or flowers on the table may perk up the appetite.

— *Plan for longer meal times*: Don't schedule activities close to meals. Don't be in a hurry to finish eating.

— *Walk before meals*: A short walk often helps stimulate appetite.

— *Stay away from unpleasant topics*: Meal times should be pleasant times and unpleasant topics may cause stress and loss of appetite.

Some Tips to Make Food Tastier:

1. Try experimenting with various foods to see whether you can find something that is satisfying.

2. If your problem is a diminishing sense of taste, try increasing the quantity of spicy foods you eat. There is no harm in adding a little pepper or even chilly if it makes food pleasant. If you don't suffer from heart problem or an excess of cholesterol, a little ghee or butter will add flavour to your food.

Food—The best way to enjoy it: If sleep takes up a third of your day, eating also takes up a good part of it. To some of us, it is the most enjoyable pleasure of all. Regular meal times become established and hunger builds up prior to these times. Our body 'clock' works with astonishing regularity. Hunger leads to ill humour and irritation and hence frequent and smaller meals are preferable to the usual one large meal each day and two smaller ones. Filling the stomach once daily with a large amount of food, or stuffing yourself causes excessive rush of blood in the abdominal vessels. A reflex provides more circulation for absorption of the products of digestion into the bloodstream. But this means less blood for your brain and muscles.

Moreover, your heart strains to provide this blood for the extra circulation. Certainly not ideal if you have a weak heart. Drowsiness and dizziness result after a heavy and big meal. When less blood is available for the muscles, the sustained effort is poor. Fatigue sets in early, so small but frequent meals will not produce this heart strain and brain deprivation.

THE PROBLEM OF WEIGHT

The western world and particularly the U.S. and Canada are experiencing an epidemic of obesity. If one travels from Asia to Europe and then to the U.S., one is amazed how obese these people have become. The disease is slowly catching on in India as well. Ours is a country full of contradictions. On one hand there are emaciated bodies afflicted by malnutrition and sometimes by semi-starvation and on the other hand, men and women visit slimming centres and spend thousands of rupees to lose a few kilograms.

As affluence increases and modern home gadgets and cars and scooters become abundant, our life is becoming less active, food becomes richer and expenditure of calories becomes less. Two inventions have added fuel to the fire. These are televisions and computers, especially personal computers. These two things draw young people into many more hours of immobility. Those above fifty are not so much affected by computers but television is making their life more slothful. The affluent class avoids walking and the fat accumulated in youth makes matters worse as age increases. People become less active and sometimes may become couch-potatoes. If the food remains the same in quality and sometimes quantity as well, it becomes a breeding ground for diseases like diabetes, hypertension, cardiovascular disease and may be arthritis. The legs become overburdened by the body weight and the knee joints may give way.

In the world, Japan is a country where obesity has been extremely uncommon. Japanese love to eat and can eat a lot but they certainly walk more and consume less fat. Moreover, they are rice eaters and rice diets have a reputation for helping people lose weight. Rice-eating cultures eat the whole grains of the plant, even if polished, whereas wheat-eating cultures eat pulverised grains, primarily in products made from flour. Cooked rice absorbs more water and the volume is more than wheat flour and hence the quantity of starch naturally comes down for rice eaters.

Losing weight has become a cultural obsession in some countries and with a section of our own society. There are lots of advertisements in newspapers and weight reduction has become an industry in itself. Magical solutions are offered and there are medicines which control hunger. But the research on this point is incomplete and the basic problem is that interference in the mechanics of energy production may lead to unforeseen, seriously adverse effects.

The basic equation that relates to calorie intake to weight is very simple. If calorie intake consistently exceeds calorie expenditure, the body will tend to store excess calories as fat. Nutritionists recommend that moderately active adults consume between 2000 and 3000 calories a day, depending on gender and body size. If you put 1500 calories or more in your breakfast with parathas, butter, sweets etc. and then have two more meals, you are sure to become an obese person.

Apart from calorie intake, certain other factors can influence the basic equation. First and foremost among these is genetics. In certain human beings there exists the so-called thrifty genes that allow some people to store up available calories as fat more readily than others. Such genes were a great advantage in populations that often faced near starvation or went through periodic cycles of feast and famine. Our distant ancestors probably lived mostly in those conditions in which these genes developed. Some people say that they gain weight by just looking at food. It may not be true but it is a fact that many of us are genetically programmed to turn available calories into fat quickly. The problem is that those genes are no longer advantageous to the people for whom food and calories are available in excess and abundance. All of us know some people who eat constantly and remain lean.

In fact, some of them want to gain weight and complain of an inability to do so. Actually they have a different sort of genetic constitution. The principal mechanism by which genes regulate hunger and body fat through an appetite control centre is the hypothelamus, a deep brain structure that regulates many body functions. In each of us, this mechanism is set to a certain point, mostly determined by genes and relatively resistant to change. The setting keeps us at a certain weight compensating for changes in activity and variations in caloric intake. This is the main reason that dieting is so frustrating. As the caloric intake is reduced, the hypothelamus turns stored fat into calories. But as soon as a normal diet is resumed, weight increases.

There are some cultural issues which surround obesity. Being fat is a major disadvantage in our cultured society. It puts you at odds with prevailing standards of beauty and attractiveness. Though all women wish to appear attractive, obesity becomes a major obstacle to it.

A Longer Life

Besides appearance, in several studies obesity was found to be associated with:

— Fifteen times greater risk of uterine cancer

— Increased risk of breast cancer

— Increased risk of heart disease

— Diabetes and blood pressure

— Higher levels of anger, anxiety and depression.

Some scientists believe that the benefits of remaining lean go beyond just preventing disease to actually slowing the process of ageing. Experiments made on animals show that dietary restrictions imposed for weight reduction also slow down the ageing process and delay the onset of age-related physiological deterioration. A diet low in calories and high in fibre helps protect cell membranes from ageing quickly.

Diet management is a problem and also an art for reducing weight. It does not mean taking two meagre meals a day. If you approach weight loss with a mindset of deprivation, you will not succeed. Instead you must find ways to eat less while managing your hunger. Hunger management is not just about taking care of physical appetite. It also includes satisfying the desire for pleasure from food in all its aspects. If you don't satisfy hunger during the day, you will find yourself eating more in the evening taking in more calories than usual.

Some practical strategies may also be tried. The sight of food in abundance stimulates overeating and hence buffet dining is disastrous for such people. You should try to avoid tempting display of food. It is doubtful whether artificial sweeteners are useful in reducing weight. Usually people add them to items in meals which are top heavy in calories and made of refined flour. Not only are these useless but may prove harmful for health in the long run.

Fasting

Abstaining from food has significant effects on the body and mind. It can make more energy available to the body, at least temporarily, because digestion requires energy. For this reason fasting at the onset of a cold can shorten its duration. Fasting can also be a technique to sharpen concentration, help you gain insight into the nature of the mind and even develop spiritual awareness. But it is not a way to lose weight. Fasting prepares the body for starvation, slowing metabolism and promoting shortage of calories as fat when eating resumes.

A Simple Way to Reduce Weight

Cutting calories is the best way of weight reduction. But when you begin to cut calories, please do not reduce your level of physical activity. Various studies have shown that long-term weight loss is best achieved when you combine exercise with dietary calorie cutting. Among other things, exercise helps you burn up those extra calories. Walking one kilometre at a fast pace will burn up nearly one hundred calories. Eating food each day in five or six small meals is also useful instead of the usual three. In that way, you will be more likely to cut your appetite.

Summary of Basic Facts about Weight

— If you consistently eat more calories than you burn, you tend to store up the excess body fat.

— Genes and heredity also determine the tendency to gain weight. Many people are programmed to gain weight whenever calories are available in abundance in the body.

— If you weigh more than you should, you must not be alarmed. Try to remain fit physically and be active. Maintain a healthy lifestyle.

— Avoid all drugs, herbs, potions and exercises that promise weight loss without changing what you eat.

— To lose weight decrease calorie intake; your calories must come 50 to 60 percent from carbohydrates, 30 percent from fat and 10 to 20 percent from proteins.

— Avoid refined sugar, and atta. Use more whole meal atta.

— Increase calorie expenditure by increasing physical activity. Isolated workouts like special exercises do little good. General activity like walking, climbing stairs, housework, gardening etc. are more effective.

— Dieting and fasting is not the answer to keeping weight down. Almost all people who diet to lose weight, regain it when they return to normal food. You will have to change long-term patterns of eating and physical activity.

Too Thin

If obesity is a health risk, being too thin is also harmful, especially so if this underweight is the result of undereating. An eating pattern with too few calories may not supply the nutrients a person needs to keep his body running normally. A lack of food energy may cause fatigue, irritability and lack of concentration. And those with poor diet may have trouble warding off infections.

For normal weight people, a layer of body fat just under the skin helps protect the body from cold. But a very thin layer of fat becomes a problem for the frail elderly.

Much has been written about weight loss but some people may need to gain weight. For some people weight gain is as hard as weight loss is for others.

Some Tips for Weight Gain

The obvious approach for weight gain is to consume more energy than your body utilises. To gain half a kilogram of body weight, you need to consume 3000 calories that your body burns. Here are some tips:

— Consume more fats if your doctor permits. Remember you have to take care of the whole of your body and not just weight.

— Choose some foods with concentrated calories: Dry fruits, canned foods with syrup, sweets, dry milk powder, cheese are the foods for you if you are not suffering from diabetes or heart trouble.

— Eat more frequently—take five or six small meals a day.

✚ Age-Wise Height and Weight Chart ✚

	Age in years	Height without shoes in cms.	Weight in kilograms	Height in inches
Male	10-12	140	35	55"
	12-14	151	43	59"
	14-18	170	59	67"
	18-22	175	67	69"
	22-35	175	70	69"
	35-55	173	70	68"
	55-75+	171	70	67"

	Age in years	Height without shoes in cms.	Weight in kilograms	Height in inches
Female	10-12	142	35	56"
	12-14	154	44	61"
	14-16	157	52	62"
	16-18	160	54	63"
	18-22	163	58	64"
	22-35	163	58	64"
	35-55	160	58	63"
	55-75+	157	58	62"

SOME OLD AGE DISEASES RELATED TO FOOD

Diseases can be of three types:

1. Diseases or disorders caused by nutrient deficiency.
2. Diseases which have several causes, some of which are food and nutrient related.
3. Diseases which have no direct food or nutrient related cause.

Giving foods and nutrients in concentrated form is effective therapy for those diseases we have mentioned in the first category/type. Food and diet play an all important role in the treatment of these disorders.

Diseases in the second category include diabetes and coronary heart diseases (CHD). Consumption of excessive amounts of sugar and refined carbohydrates can precipitate diabetes in individuals who are already genetically predisposed. Similarly, consumption of diets containing excessive amounts of fats, particularly saturated fats and cholesterol, is believed to be a cause of CHD and the underlying process of narrowing of arteries by deposition of fat (atherosclerosis).

In the case of these diseases, diet alone cannot cure disease, it can only help to check the progress of the disease and also to prevent complications. Diet therapy, therefore, helps patients lead a full life. Without it, the disease can become uncontrollable irrespective of whether the patient is also prescribed drugs or not. In fact, mild cases can be controlled by diet alone.

Infectious diseases are good examples of the third category. Some of these may be transmitted through food. However, food is not the direct cause. Treatment of these diseases usually does include a greater or lesser degree of diet therapy. For example, a febrile infectious disease (disease associated with fever) would require giving the patient additional energy- and protein-rich foods in a suitable form. This would depend on whether the fever is chronic, as in the case of tuberculosis, or acute, as in typhoid.

Here are some diseases which are related to the first and second category. These can afflict a person of any age but elders past fifty are more prone to these ailments.

High Blood Pressure

High blood pressure or hypertension means higher than normal pressure on blood vessel walls. It occurs as blood gets pushed through small blood vessels that have become stiff and narrow. High blood pressure causes the heart to work harder and over time may damage artery walls. Damage to blood vessels in the brain may cause a stroke.

To correct a misconception, hypertension is not the same as emotional tension or stress, although stress may temporarily raise blood pressure levels. Even people who are calm and relaxed can have high blood pressure.

Causes of High Blood Pressure:

— **Heredity:** People appear to have a hereditary tendency for blood pressure. If your parents have hypertension, there are chances that you will also develop it.

— **Overweight:** Extra body fat, especially around the waste and midriff, increases the risk for high blood pressure.

— **Age factor:** For many people, blood pressure goes up as they get older. For men it is sooner, perhaps starting by age 45 to 50. In women, it often starts 7 to 10 years later. They become susceptible after menopause.

— **Inactive lifestyle:** Sedentary living does not cause high blood pressure and physical activity alone won't bring it down. But it has some effect as part of an overall lifestyle that projects against high blood pressure and heart disease.

— **Sodium sensitive:** For a large part of the population, specially those over forty, consumption of salt may contribute to high blood pressure.

— **Alcohol and smoking:** Heavy drinking and smoking increase the risk of blood pressure.

— **Some types of jobs:** Marketing executives, personal secretaries, stock brokers, and nurses are likely to develop blood pressure because of their job conditions. The first category is always under stress when sales targets are not achieved and personal secretaries have their B.P. sky-rocket when they are yelled at. Stock brokers are affected when they trade in a sliding market and the nurses when they attend a complicated operation.

Importance of Diet in the Prevention of Hypertension

Apart from regular exercise, cutting out smoking and reducing mental stress, diet is deeply involved in problems with hypertension. First, obesity can contribute to high blood pressure. So attempts should be made immediately to get rid of any excess weight. Second, reducing the intake of salt can help lower blood pressure for many people. A great number of studies have associated the sodium in salt with high blood pressure. So if you have a family history of high B.P., you should avoid adding too much salt to your foods, either during cooking or during meals. In particular, avoid potato chips, pickles, biscuits, sauces, fast foods, frozen peas etc.

It is also recommended that the intake of fibre in diet should be increased. This means eating more whole grains, brans, vegetables and pules.

The intake of fruits like apples, guavas, melons, oranges, etc. should be increased. Vegetables like beans, cabbages, cauliflowers, peas, boiled potatoes, radishes are also useful.

As stated above, hypertension patients benefit from diets low in sodium. The normal diet contains about 3 to 6 gms. of sodium. Low sodium diet ranges from 200 to 300 mg. right up to 2000-3000 mg depending on the degree of restriction. Liver and kidney disorders and cardiac failure also need low sodium diet.

This chart specifies the level of sodium prescribed for different types of disorders.

Degree of sodium restriction	Level of sodium permitted	Description of diet	Disease condition
Extreme	200-300 mg	No salt in cooking. Selection of very low sodium-containing foods.	Cirrhosis of liver with ascites; severe congestive heart failure.
Severe	500-700 mg	No salt in cooking. Selection of low-sodium foods.	Severe congestive heart failure. Severe renal disease with oedema in patients not on dialysis; cirrhosis with ascites (fluid in abdomen).
Moderate	1000-1500 mg	No salt in cooking; measured amounts of salt, salted bread and butter.	Strong family history of hypertension or patients with borderline hypertension.

Contd...

Degree of sodium restriction	Level of sodium permitted	Description of diet	Disease condition
Mild	2000-3000 mg	Some amount of salt can be used in cooking but no salty food permitted, no salt to be used at table.	Maintenance diet in cardiac and renal diseases.

Diabetes

Diabetes affects more than 5 crore people in India and the number may rise to 10 crores in the next two decades. It affects both young and the elderly but age is a prominent factor in this disease.

On its own, diabetes can have serious, even life-threatening, effects on health. It is also a risk factor for other health problems. Heart disease, eye problems, foot problem and kidney disease are among the many conditions related to diabetes.

What is Diabetes:

Simply defined, diabetes is a condition that affects the way the body uses energy in food.

During digestion, glucose, a form of sugar, is released from carbohydrates in food. Once absorbed into the blood, it is referred to as blood glucose, or blood sugar. Among healthy people, insulin, made in the pancreas, regulates blood sugar levels. It allows glucose to pass into your body cells where it is changed to energy. And it helps your body use amino acids and fatty acids from food.

People with diabetes have trouble controlling their blood sugar, or blood glucose levels. In such people the body does not produce enough insulin or can't use it properly. As a result, the body cannot use energy nutrients—carbohydrates, proteins and fats in their normal way. Glucose accumulates in blood, causing blood sugar levels to rise. Rather than being used for energy, blood sugar passes out of the body through urine. That makes extra work for the kidneys, causing frequent urination and excessive thirst.

Actually there are three types of diabetes:

1. Type I (insulin dependent) is less common. It happens when the pancreas cannot make insulin or at least not enough. Often this type of diabetes begins in childhood or the young adult years. But people of any age can get it.

2. Type II (non-insulin dependent) diabetes is more common. Typically it runs in families. It is a disease that develops slowly and usually becomes evident after age 40.

3. Gestational diabetes occurs during pregnancy as a result of changes in hormone levels. Usually it disappears after the baby is born.

Here we are more concerned with type II or non-insulin dependent diabetes. If you have two or more of these risk factors, your chances are higher:

■ Over age 40.

■ Close family members with diabetes.

■ More than 20 percent over the weight that is healthy for you.

■ Have high blood pressure or high blood cholesterol.

■ A lethargic lifestyle, lack of exercise combined with intake of fatty foods.

■ Excessive consumption of some types of medicines like antibiotics, diuretics, steroids.

■ Lack of some nutrients in food like chromium, lime, Vitamin E.

■ Some major accident or surgery.

■ Excessive stress, tension, or depression.

Symptoms: Frequent urination, excessive hunger and thirst are the initial symptoms. Rapid reduction in weight without any apparent cause and a feeling of weakness and exhaustion may follow later on. Vision may also become weak and glasses have to be changed frequently. A cut does not heal for a long time. This is also a symptom of this disease.

Early detection: Early detection of the disease is very important. Diabetes can be easily detected by blood and urine test. It is advisable that everyone aged 50 or over should have a blood glucose test every alternate year.

Control: Diabetes can be controlled by four measures: Having knowledge about diabetes and the ability to undertake tests yourself, a balanced diet, exercise and medicines.

If diabetes strikes you, there is no need to be nervous and puzzled. Books are available on the subject and knowing more about it will enable you to face it with more confidence.

Diet and exercise: Everyone who has diabetes needs to follow an eating plan and a physical activity plan too. For some people, weight loss and active living are enough to control their blood sugar levels and maintain good health. For others, pills or injections also may be needed to keep blood sugar levels under control.

In the early years of diabetes, you can do the most to protect your body from the long-term hazards of this disease. If your blood sugar level is high for long periods of time over many years, diabetes may cause major damage to your nervous system and to the blood vessels in your eyes, kidneys, heart and feet. The good news is you can prevent or reduce this damage. In turn, you may live longer with fewer problems.

Eating plan: If you have diabetes, there is no single way to eat. The proportions of carbohydrates, protein and fat in your eating plan depend on you, including your weight, blood cholesterol level, and medical needs. What you eat also depends on what foods you enjoy. In the past, a strictly planned diet for diabetes prescribed specific ratios for energy nutrients, carbohydrates, protein and fat. Recently the guidelines have become more flexible to meet individual needs. Actually a diabetic diet is not too different from any healthy eating pattern. That is especially true for people with non-insulin dependent diabetes.

Some Fallacies Regarding Food for Diabetics:

- **Sugar alone causes diabetes:** Experts now know that starches and rice, bread, potato and fruits and vegetables containing carbohydrate and sugar have a similar effect on blood sugar levels. Actually, sugar does not cause blood sugar levels to rise any more rapidly than starches do. So people with diabetes can have sugary foods in moderation. The total amount of carbohydrates is the issue, not just the quantity of sugar.

- **Chewing neem or some bitter thing will cure diabetes:** Chewing neem leaves or some other thing having bitter taste does not cure diabetes. The fact is that the bitter taste makes the taste buds on the tongue inactive for some time which produces an aversion for food. Thus, the consumption of less food naturally leads to lower blood sugar level. In the long run, it may lead to malnutrition. Of course, there are some herbs which lower blood sugar level, but it is not necessary that they taste bitter.

- **Drinking of water kept in a copper pot cures the disease:** Drinking of water cures constipation and one feels good. If one drinks water frequently, the intake for food is decreased, which leads to a lower blood sugar level.

- **Mere medicines will cure the disease and no control on diet or physical exercise is required:** Keeping your blood sugar at a steady level means you need to have regular 'refuelling'. Skipping meals, eating at different times and taking too much carbohydrates are damaging and medicine alone will not be able to control the consequences.

Regular physical activity is an important part of managing diabetes. Physical activity helps your body transport glucose to body cells, and results in a lower level of blood sugar by using calories. It also reduces the risk of heart disease which is linked to diabetes.

- **Crash dieting to control weight is dangerous:** If you are overweight, try to control it by reducing fats and carbohydrates in your food gradually and in a safe manner. It will be better to take the advice of a physician or dietician. But total stoppage of the above may lead to serious consequences. Your blood sugar level may go down to a dangerous level and may lead to coma.

- **Sweet fruits are not always harmful:** The sweetness or sourness of a fruit is not a measure of its calorie value. Water melon is very sweet but contains only 16 calories whereas a raw mango, though sour in taste, has 90 calories. Not eating any fruit at all is harmful and may lead to anaemia, night blindness, and such other diseases produced by the lack of vitamins and minerals. Of course, mango, banana, grapes etc. should be taken occasionally while other fruits should be taken regularly.

- **Raw or half-baked food is beneficial:** Boiling or baking the food does not alter its calorie value. People living in villages usually do not suffer from diabetes not because they take raw or half-boiled food but because they are always on the move, do more physical work and have less mental tension.

As stated above, diet is a centre pillar in therapy for diabetes. The goals for dietary management of diabetes are to:

— Improve the overall health of the patient by attaining and maintaining optimum nutrition.

— Attain and maintain ideal body weight.

— Maintain blood glucose as near the normal physiological range as possible.

— Prevent or delay development of chronic complications of diabetes—cardiovascular, renal, retinal and neurological.

— Modify the diet as required for treating and preventing complications of diabetes and associated diseases.

In a nutshell, the salient features of diet for diabetes are:

— Attainment and maintenance of desirable body weight according to age, sex, activity level; intake of complex carbohydrates (starches) rather than simple carbohydrates (sugars); high-fibre content in the diet and intake of polyunsaturated fats in preference to saturated fats.

Here are some diabetic diets with specific points to remember according to the guidelines for standardised hospital diets laid down by the Director General of Health Services.

	1200 Kcal	1500 Kcal	1800 Kcal	2000 Kcal	2500 Kcal
Cereals	125 g	175 g	225 g	225 g	350 g
Pulses	50 g	50 g	50 g	75 g	75 g
Milk and Milk Products	500 ml	500 ml	750 ml	750 ml	750 ml
Green Vegetables	200 g	200 g	200 g	200 g	200 g
Other Vegetables	200 g	200 g	200 g	200 g	200 g
Fruits	1 portion	1 portion	1 portion	1 portion	2 portions
Paneer/Egg	30 g/one	30 g/one	30 g/one	30 g/one	30 g/one
Oil	10 g	15 g	15 g	20 g	25 g
Sugar	–	–	–	–	–

Foods Allowed Liberally

Green leafy vegetables, vegetable salads without oil dressings, lime, lemonade soups.

Note:

1. Roasted Bengal gram and fenugreek seeds can be included in the diet as these have been shown to have a hypoglycaemic effect.

2. One portion of fruit providing 10 gm carbohydrate.

Black coffee or tea without milk or with day's allowance.

Chutneys and pickles without oil.

Pepper and jeera water

Jamun, phalsa, raspberry.

Foods to Avoid

Soft drinks, all beverages not listed above.

Alcohol and wines.

Fried foods.

Sugar, honey, jams, sweets, cakes, pastries.

Heart Disease

In India we are in the midst of a heart disease epidemic and about four people die of heart attack every minute. Two factors account for this upsurge of heart disease: Genetic factors and new-found prosperity for a section of the Indian population. A ten-year study of 4500 patients was made by the Coronary Artery Disease Institute (CADI) in Listle, Illinois, U.S.A. The researchers came to the conclusion that the Indian community has much higher levels of a deadly

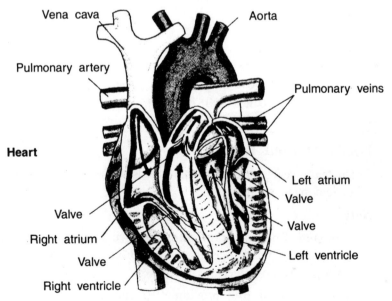

genetic factor called Lipoproteins (a) than other ethnic groups. It is 10 times deadlier in causing clogged arteries that lead to heart attacks than bad cholesterol such as Low Density Lipoproteins (LDL). This factor, called *Cardiac syndrome X* by specialists, leaves Indians four times more prone to heart disease than Chinese, Japanese, Caucasians and Hispanics.

However, all physicians do not agree with this theory. They are of the opinion that the genes load the gun, lifestyle pulls the trigger. Lifestyle changes, due to rapid urbanisation, are precipitating the cause of heart disease. While over 10 percent of urban Indians succumb to heart disease, the figure is only 3.5 percent in rural areas. Actually undetected diabetics, hypertension, a fat-rich diet, heavy smoking, lack of exercise and late detection are all recipes for disaster.

Of those who suffer from heart disease, only twenty-five percent are below forty years of age and the rest are above forty and mostly above fifty.

Diet is one of the several factors which is believed to cause cardiovascular problems (heart disease). As the process of the disease starts, fatty substances such as cholesterol compounds called esters, cholesterol and triglycerides are deposited on inside walls of arteries. The deposit grows till it partially or completely blocks the artery. This process is called atherosclerosis and is responsible for heart disease and even strokes (paralysis).

Generally, diet therapy for these and other types of cardiovascular disorders is based on four simple rules.

1. Give the patients only the amount of food which would maintain weight. Putting on extra weight is dangerous. If the patient is overweight, a low calorie diet should be taken.

2. Plan the menu around those foods that are easy to digest.

3. Restrict stimulants such as tea, coffee, cocoa.

4. Limit salt. If oedema is present, restrict sodium intake substantially.

The patient should also:

— Give the heart a much needed rest.

— Prevent or eliminate accumulation of fluid in the body i.e. oedema.

— Maintain good nutrition.

Obesity and overweight mean bad news for heart patients. There are three reasons why the cardiac patient should not be obese:

— The heart must work harder as the body pushes and pulls the extra weight around.

— Fat deposits in the myocardium decrease efficiency of these muscles.

— Abdominal fat interferes with movement of the diaphragm and thus free action of the heart.

In the acute phase of heart disease, the following diet is recommended. Although these diets have been approved by the Director General of Health Services, the physician or dietician should still be consulted before going on such a diet.

(a) 1000 Kcal liquid diet

Milk and milk products (curd etc.)	730 ml
Egg white	One
Fruits for juice	200 g
Vegetables for soup	200 g
Cereal (for porridges, bread)	150 g
Sugar	20 g
Oil (unsaturated)	10 g

This is a diet which is:

— Low cholesterol

— Low fat

— Sodium restricted

— Low calorie.

To reduce stress on the body system, it is desirable to give frequent liquid feeds.

In severe myocardial infraction the following diet schedule may be adopted:

1-3 days: Clear fluid diet consisting of fruit juice, coconut water and barley water containing glucose.

3-6 days: 800 ml milk given in four equal feeds i.e. 200 ml every 4 hours (provided the patient can tolerate milk and has no abdominal distension).

7-10 days: Semi-liquid diet providing 800-1000 Kcal.

11-14 days: Semi-solid diet providing 1200 Kcal.

The above diet is suitable once the patient's condition has stabilised somewhat and the initial phase is over. As the patient improves, he is put on a maintenance diet.

(b) Maintenance diet-1800 Kcal.

Milk and milk products	750 g
Egg white	One
Paneer/Meat/Chicken	30/50 g
Fruit	200 g
Dal	25 g
Vegetables	400 g
Cereal	200 g
Sugar	20 g
Oil (unsaturated)	15 g

Care has to be taken to omit salt and foods in which salt or baking powder has been added.

Once the patient returns home he or she has to take special care in keeping the diet low in fat and if problems persist, sodium as well. Total intake of calories should be restricted according to need. Cholesterol sources, such as egg yolk and glandular meats, are not permitted as the following list tells you:

97

Foods not permitted:

— Glandular meat e.g. kidney, liver, brain.

— Whole milk, cream, ice-cream, khoa and other preparations made of whole milk.

— Butter, ghee, hydrogenated fat, coconut oil, palm oil.

— Egg yolk, processed cheese.

— Sweets of all kinds, cakes, pastries.

— Dry nuts like almonds, walnut, groundnut, coconut.

— Fried foods.

— Cocoa and chocolate-based drinks.

— All aerated waters.

— Alcohol-based beverages and other products.

— High-sodium foods (if there is oedema) e.g. bread, biscuits, eggs, cakes, pastries, canned vegetables, soups and fruits, salted or smoked fish, chicken, cheese, salted nuts, peanut butter, salted pickles, samosas, and other savoury preparations.

Cancer

After heart disease and diabetes, cancer is also emerging in India as a leading cause of illness and death. Among men, the incidence of prostate cancer is very high followed by lung cancer. In women, breast cancer is the highest. Recently, in some regions, mouth cancer is also raging due to the habit of chewing tobacco and pan masala.

Cancer is more than one disease. But they all have characteristics in common: abnormal cell growth that spreads and destroys other organs and body tissues. Cancers are classified by the body tissues where the cancer starts, such as colon, breast or skin.

Cancer starts with a single cell that gets out of control. An altered body cell multiplies at an abnormally fast rate. Because they are abnormal, they no longer function normally. Yet, they use the body's resources, including nutrients, to multiply. In the process, they disrupt and eventually destroy the normal function of tissue or organ where they grow gradually. These cancerous cells spread to other parts of the body, invading and destroying healthy body tissues and organs.

Cancer risk increases with age: Recently, a number of studies have focussed on the body's immune system, with its defence mechanism against cancer. It has been estimated that the disease doubles its incidence for every decade past thirty. The older people get, the more likely they are to get cancer. The reason may be that the body's immune system, which enables it to fight many threats, shows a decline with age. One more reason may be that the cancer virus, lying dormant for many years, flares up. Tobacco, which is known to be weakly cancer producing, shows its effect after a long period of time. The slowness of the development of the disease may be the chief reason for the apparent link between ageing and cancer.

Cancer of the prostate also comes on fairly late in life. It rarely emerges before a man is in his fifties, but then it rises to become perhaps the most common cancer in men in their seventies and beyond. Hence, it has been nicknamed 'the old man's cancer'.

Nutritious ways to reduce cancer risk: The relationship between nutrition and cancer is not as clear as nutrition's link to heart disease. But in a majority of deaths due to cancer, diet plays a prominent role. So while planning a diet, keep the following facts in mind:

1. High-fat diets have been definitely implicated in an increased incidence of cancer of the breast and the bowel. Vegetables and fruits have a complex composition with more than 100 vitamins, minerals, fibre and other substances, which may offer protection from cancer.

2. Some Vitamin A components of the diet seem to lower the incidence of cancer. These nutrients are found in green vegetables, fruits and fruit juices.

3. There are certain other foods that seem to have special protective values. Certain vegetables (cauliflower, sprouted grains) have been shown to diminish the cancer of intestinal tract.

4. Obesity leads an individual to cancer. So a diet suitable for reduction in obesity also prevents the disease.

5. Food items containing Vitamin C and E are also useful in the prevention of cancer.

6. Last of all, heavy drinking leads to liver cancer and smoking enhances the chance of mouth, throat and larynx cancer.

Constipation

Constipation is often defined with two characteristics in mind: (1) a condition in which stool or faecal matter in the intestines is hard to pass in an attempted bowel movement, and (2) a dissatisfaction with the size and adequacy of the bowel movements.

Many times, constipation is thought of with only the physical problems in mind. So we may focus on the facts that the faeces in constipated bowels tend to be smaller and drier than usual, and that one person may go to the toilet less frequently than normal. But "regularity" is a relative concept. Some people are having healthy, regular bowel movements if they take two trips to the toilet each day. Others are regular if they go every other day.

In any case, your feelings about your bowels are important because only you know what sort of bowel pattern makes you feel satisfied and relaxed. Sometimes, those who have "regular" daily bowel movements still suffer from a form of constipation. The reason for this is that the rectum may not be completely emptied after a bowel movement because of the presence of hard or dry faecal matter. If a relatively large amount of faeces remains in your intestines, you may still feel slow, sluggish, uncomfortable or out-of-sorts, even after you have had a bowel movement.

Very often we tend to think of constipation as an inevitable consequence of growing older. But everyone regardless of age gets constipated some time or the other. It is true that an ageing colon loses some muscle tone. It is also true that the wave-like contractions in the colon—the motion that pushes waste through the system—grow a bit sluggish. But the colon, like the rest of the digestive tract, was designed to function adequately even when not operating at peak performance.

Besides this change in the body, there are other contributing factors to constipation:

■ **A failure to include sufficient amounts of cellulose fibre and other bulk in the diet:** Every person's diet, and especially that of those in the second half of life, should include plenty of fruits and vegetables. These foods contain plenty of bulk, or fibrous material that swells in the intestines and facilitates bowel movements. Bran of cereals also contains a great deal of helpful fibre.

On the other hand, it is important not to overdo consumption of bran. Those who eat excessive amounts—which may be defined generally as more than one normal-size cereal bowl per day—may start eliminating too many important nutrients through their stools. For example, extended and excessive use of wheat bran or even isafgol bran has been shown to produce reduced levels of iron and calcium in the blood.

■ **A tendency to eat too many foods that cause constipation:** For some people, processed cheese may encourage hard stools. Others may respond similarly to foods that are high in animal fats, such as meats, milk and other dairy products, and eggs. The same may be true of many refined sugary foods, fried foods, sweets etc.

101

The simple solution to this problem is to reduce or eliminate these foods from your diet and to substitute more high-fibre products.

■ **A failure to drink enough water and other liquids:** Everyone should drink at least ten glasses of water per day, or the equivalent in easily digestible juices. In addition, the older people who have problems with constipation, may drink a glass of warm to hot water in the morning adding a little lemon juice. This liquid frequently initiates a wave of activity in the intestines that can end with satisfactory results.

■ **A failure to use natural food laxatives:** Many times, in addition to bran, foods such as guavas, papayas, apples, can trigger a bowel movement. You can learn best what works for you by experimenting.

■ **A failure to respond when the urge strikes:** When you feel that you need to have a bowel movement, that is the time to head for the toilet. If you delay or procrastinate, the urge may pass, and the likelihood will increase that part of your stool will harden and create constipation problems.

■ **A failure to exercise regularly:** Exercise helps combat constipation in several important ways. First, the movement of your body during exercise helps to soften and break up faecal matter in your intestines.

Second, one of the reasons that people become constipated as they grow older is that, as do other parts of the body, the muscles that are involved in bowel movements, grow weaker with age. Specifically, the muscles of the diaphragm, abdominal wall, and pelvic floor lose their power to cause the expulsive force that pushes a stool out of the body.

A general physical-fitness regimen, with an emphasis on abdominal and mid-body strengthening, stretching, and conditioning, can do wonders for maintaining the power and tone of some of the muscles that help expedite bowel movements.

- **Abuse of laxatives or enemas:** Our first reaction to constipation is to run to the drug store for a laxative. It is wrong. Laxatives may actually cause constipation rather than remedy it. At best, they temporarily solve a problem that demands a long-term cure. Instead, our first reaction should be to increase fibre in our diet. There is widespread agreement among doctors and researchers that dietary fibre (especially bran) is a safe and effective way of guarding against constipation.

  Those who depend on laxatives are teaching their colons to be lazy. After relying on such products, the colon can "forget" how to function on its own. In other words, frequent laxative use can actually cause constipation.

  Doctors suggest adding fibre to the diet and increasing exercise to combat irregularity. If you need to take a laxative, they say, use it sparingly and choose a gentle product rather than a stimulant formula. Gentle laxatives work by increasing the bulk in the colon or softening stool by causing the colon to retain fluid.

A variety of other factors may also contribute to constipation such as:

- Uncomfortable or unpleasant toilet facilities; like an arthritic patient using an Indian-type toilet.
- Changes of environment; a long rail or bus journey.
- Emotional or physical stress.
- Drugs such as antidepressants, antacids containing aluminium or calcium and diuretics.
- Depression or mental confusion; or
- Failure to develop basic bowel-movement habits at a younger age.

Many times, you can correct these problems and develop a regular, healthy routine of bowel movements with preventive measures, such as good nutrition. Despite all that I have said above, old people may need the help of drugs or other laxatives or enemas. As long as these substances or procedures are not abused, they can be quite helpful in overcoming constipation. But any extended use of these methods should only be tried with a doctor's advice.

Gas

Many people suffer from gaseous trouble and numerous medicines are available claiming to combat the malady. Although anyone who swallows either air or food gets gas, it seems to trouble the young and the ageing more rather than the in-betweens. Babies are gas-prone because they swallow air as they drink from the bottle or breast. People in their 20s and 30s have problems because of poor eating habits, nervous temperaments and lactose (milk sugar) intolerance.

We may blame stabbing gas pains on the spicy and fatty foods, but doctors say that two-thirds of the gas in most people's systems is simply swallowed air. Fast eaters, straw sippers, cold sufferers and tea and coffee gulpers are good candidates for stomach gas caused by swallowed air. And because some air is swallowed each time saliva goes down, habits that make the mouth water, like chewing gum, smoking and sucking mints, can also cause gas. Carbonated beverages are an obvious hazard.

Talking with a full mouth, chewing with an open mouth, slurping hot tea—our punishment may be painful stomach gas and its socially unacceptable counterpart: the belch. The best defence is a relaxed meal-time atmosphere.

The gas that isn't caused by swallowed air is the natural by-product of the breakdown of foods in the gastrointestinal tract. Ordinarily our stomach holds about three ounces of gas, disposing of it inconspicuously by absorption into the bloodstream. The problem arises when the foods we eat produce too much gas. Foods rich in complex carbohydrates like beans, bran, cauliflower and cabbage tend to be the biggest gas producers. Other common offenders are: bananas, popcorn, onions, peanuts, coffee and chocolate. Inadequate carbohydrate absorption is fermented by bacteria in the large intestine to produce gases such as carbon dioxide, hydrogen, methane and oxygen.

Sometimes, middle-aged persons may not tolerate milk. The reason is that the production of lactose—(the crizyone needed to digest milk sugar) slows in many people as they age. Gas is a major symptom of milk intolerance. If you are so affected, avoid dairy products like yoghurt, cheese or sweets made of milk. Your physician can also help you by prescribing lactose products when taking milk.

Haemorrhoids (Piles)

The appearance of the unpleasant condition known as 'haemorrhoids' is often associated with straining during constipation and by implication with an improper diet.

A haemorrhoid is simply a distended little vein covered with overlying tissue, which appears either at the anal opening or just inside the anal canal. The first is called an external haemorrhoid, and the second is known as an internal haemorrhoid.

You can easily feel external haemorrhoids, which are usually about the size of a pea. Several of them may appear together and form an encircling cluster. People usually learn they have haemorrhoids when the surface of the haemorrhoid is torn and bleeding results or simply when pain or discomfort occurs in the anal areas.

Sometimes, haemorrhoids may become so bothersome that your doctor may recommend surgical removal. When internal haemorrhoids begin to protrude, it may be possible to reduce pain by tucking them back inside the rectum.

Another possibility for treating haemorrhoids is the use of laser beams. The lasers destroy the tissue, coagulate the blood, and cause the haemorrhoids to fall off. This procedure is usually performed on an outpatient basis. The patient gets admitted in a hospital for a few hours to undergo the surgery by a specialist known as a proctologist and then is released from the hospital the same day. The laser has similarly been used for treatment of fissures (painful cracks at the anal opening) that may or may not be associated with haemorrhoids.

In most cases, however, minor haemorrhoid symptoms can be relieved simply by taking a hot sitz bath (a bath taken in around six inches of water while sitting) or by applying soothing anaesthetic ointments. Many of these products can be bought over the counter.

Because constipation may trigger problems with haemorrhoids, one line of attack against this problem may be to pay more attention to your diet. Among other steps, you should consider making the dietary changes that are necessary to eliminate the constipation, and then the haemorrhoids will often take care of themselves.

But before you try to treat yourself, it is best to check with your doctor. Sometimes, haemorrhoids are associated with other disorders higher up in the rectum or colon, and only a physician can be sure that they are the result of common, less risky causes such as constipation.

Heartburn

Heartburn has nothing to do with the heart—although its intense chest pain may scare you into thinking you are having a heart attack. And, contrary to general belief, it's not a stomach disorder. It's actually an inflammation of the food pipe caused when stomach acid backs up through the muscular valve between the stomach and food pipe. Unlike the stomach, the food pipe has no mucous lining to protect it from gastric acids.

Normally, the valve opens to allow food into the stomach while keeping stomach contents from flowing back up and acting on the bare walls of the food pipe. But a number of things can cause the system to go awry. Overeating can cause abdominal pressure to relax the valve. Certain foods like chocolates, fats, oils, and carbonated beverages can also lessen the tension of the valve. Nicotine and alcohol have similar effects. Hearty partying, which may combine several overindulgences, is, thus, a prime cause of heartburn.

Air swallowers may also experience heartburn when their bloated stomach increases pressure on the food pipe valve, so may pregnant women when an expanding uterus pushes against the stomach and releases the valve. Lifestyle may be a factor too. Stress and tension stimulate the flow of gastric juices. Eating on the run or eating while working often means poorly chewed food, an overworked stomach and increased abdominal pressure.

The fastest cure for heartburn is a few swallows of water or food—anything that washes away the irritating acid in the food pipe. Antacids may also provide relief by neutralising stomach juices. But the only permanent cure comes from changing eating and lifestyle habits.

Ulcers

They were once thought to be an 'executive ailment', dues extracted from the corporate ladder-climber on the way to a vice-presidency and a posher suburb. But now researchers say there is no evidence that ulcers strike those in any particular occupations or social or financial strata.

It is true that some people—irrespective of career or bank book—react strongly to stress by producing excess gastric acid. Over time, this may eat away at the lining of the stomach or duodenum (the first section of the small intestine) causing painful sores known as ulcers. Coffee, alcohol, aspirin and hurried eating habits also increase acid production. Some people may be predisposed to ulcers because of a thinner, less protective gut lining. Another theory suggests that those with type O blood group are, for reasons not yet known, more susceptible.

Gallstones

A disease of the overfed or the genetically unlucky, gallstones are hardened masses of cholesterol, blood and bile salts.

Sometimes microscopic, sometimes as big as oversized marbles, the stones form in the gall-bladder or the bile duct leading from the gall-bladder to the small intestines.

Although no one knows exactly why far more women suffer from gallstones than men, one theory is that those who frequently gain and lose large amounts of weight—as women do during pregnancy—are more susceptible. Studies have shown that gallstones are twice as common in women over 40 as in middle-aged men and that female vegetarians are two-and-a-half times less likely than other women to develop them. Also gallstones are more common in overweight than normal weight women and the risk increases with age.

Fortunately, as many as 75 percent of those with gallstones experience no symptoms and require no treatment. The stones may float harmlessly in the gall-bladder. Small stones may pass uneventfully through the bile duct into the small intestines and out of the body. But for the 25 percent who do suffer, the symptoms are not pleasant. Gall-bladder attacks are notoriously painful and may be accompanied by chills, fever, vomiting and jaundice. Others may suffer long-term abdominal discomfort, indigestion and nausea.

Although gallstones are associated with growing older, once again, age is not the culprit, good living is. Scientists have found that a high-calorie diet is linked to increased amounts of cholesterol in the bile and to the formation of gallstones. Total calories—not the cholesterol in the diet (which has little relationship to the cholesterol in bile)—are to blame. Obviously the best hedge against this potentially gut-wrenching problem is a moderate diet that allows you to maintain normal weight.

For those who do develop gallstones and suffer acute or long-term attacks, doctors usually recommend surgical removal of the gall-bladder. A less harrowing but so far less successful treatment makes use of cholesterol-dissolving drugs. A newer, still experimental treatment uses shock waves to pulverise gallstones.

Osteoporosis

Osteoporosis is a condition of gradually weakening, brittle bones. As bones lose calcium and other minerals, they become more fragile and porous. And they may break under normal use or from just a minor fall. Because it progresses slowly and silently, people often don't realise they have osteoporosis until they fracture a bone. The spine, hip and wrist are the most common places for fractures.

Usually the signs of osteoporosis don't show up until later (usually age 60 or later). Among older adults, vertebrae in the spine compress as a result of bone loss. Such people gradually lose height and may develop back pain and disabilities.

Some factors tend to put a person at relatively high risk for osteoporosis.

— Ageing.

— Light body build or thinness.

— Female sex with early menopause.

— No exercise, immobility and little activity.

— Inadequate calcium intake.

Prevention: You cannot reverse your age or change the sex—but you can take regular exercise, and increase your mobility and work activity. The second important thing, which you can do, is to close the calcium gap. As an adult, you need plenty of calcium. If you regularly drink milk, chances are that you are getting adequate quantity of calcium. Vitamin D helps deposit calcium in bones. Try to get a little sunshine, which is not very difficult in India. In addition to milk, cheese, yoghurt and even good ice-cream are good sources. If these prove inadequate, you can take calcium pills under advice from a doctor.

Loss of Teeth

Food and teeth have a strange relationship. Bad food and bad teeth are the cause and the effect. Of course, tooth decay does not depend solely on sugary or starchy food. Whether or not you get cavities depends on many factors—and not diet alone. Heredity as well as the make up and flow of saliva are other factors. Starchy and sugary food alongwith other factors leads to tooth decay. When teeth are gone, food loses its taste. Many food items become unchewable and without proper grinding of food, indigestion becomes a problem.

Unlike other body organs, teeth are unforgiving. They don't mend themselves like bones, clean themselves like eyes, heal themselves like skin or grow out like nails. They are not only a decoration piece to make our smile perfect. They cut and grind food and mix it with saliva which is the first but very essential step in the digestive process.

Changes with Age

With the passage of time, teeth also undergo some unpleasant changes as is the case with hair, ears and eyes. As the years pass, the bright, white enamel coating thins and the darker underneath layer shows through. Deposits cause the gums to swell, redden, bleed and pull away from the teeth allowing the plaque to penetrate deeper. The cycle continues and gums continue to recede. The bacteria attack the area exposed by the receding gums. If untreated, gum disease causes teeth to loosen and fall out. But this ravage of hardened bacteria is preventable. Brush, floss and seeing the dentist regularly are the key to prevention. The key to effective brushing is a proper technique. Place the bristle at a 45-degree angle to the teeth so that they can slide beneath the gum line and get at the plaque. The brush should move on the upper jaw in a downward direction while on the lower jaw, it should be an upward movement. Brushing the teeth with a *datun*, a twig of Neem or Keeker, has its importance as it kills bacteria and strengthens gums. But for thorough cleaning, a good, soft brush is required. Even a thorough cleaning will not completely prevent the formation of plaque. Once in a while, professional cleaning should be done through a dentist.

Accumulated food, beverages and tobacco show their effect and discolour teeth. They wear away but the rate of wear is so slow that normally they can serve us for three life spans. Plaque, the invisible film of live bacteria that coats our teeth and gums, tends to accumulate faster with age causing gum inflammation. Teeth may become loose and unstable in their sockets due to loss of density of the jawbone. Gum diseases may result in minor gum bleeding or, in severe cases, in major tooth loss.

Cavities, gum disease and plaque are the villains in the drama of tooth loss. Plaque is a gummy, bacterial coating found in everyone's mouth that accumulates on teeth beneath the gum line, where it is difficult to remove. If it is not removed daily, the bacteria grow, colonise and harden into calcified clusters when they die.

Preventing Cavities

Cavities are the creation of a bacterium which ferments in the mouth when we eat sugar, resulting in an acid which eats away tooth enamel. Cavities in the teeth, when combined with gum disease, play havoc. Plaque exposes new areas of tooth decay, which may result in tooth loss and finally a false tooth. Sugar is the worst enemy of teeth, and sugar has many forms; from candies and sweets to fructose found in fruits. When you eat sugary foods and preparations that remain in your mouth for a long time, such as chocolates, hard candies, cough drops, etc. they prolong the acid attack on teeth. Sipping sweet drinks, sweet tea, soft drinks etc. frequently expose teeth to a constant sugar bath, a process that will invariably lead to tooth decay. But eating sugary foods between meals is not so harmful since the presence of other foods in the mouth mitigates the action of sugar.

Importance of Food

As in the case of many diseases and bad health conditions, food plays an important part in the preservation of teeth for a long time. Leafy green vegetables, fruits and other foods, high in Vitamin C keep gums healthy and help fight bacteria.

Milk, yoghurt and cheese are high in calcium and keep the jawbones and teeth strong and dense. Germinated grains, bran and peanuts act as buffers against mouth acid. Foods high in acids also destroy tooth enamel. Cola drinks and fruits juices are particularly harmful because they combine high acid content with high sugar levels and are often sipped over a long period of time. It is far better to eat a whole fruit than its juice because juices are more acidic. Juices also do not contain the fibrous contents of the fruit which stimulate the flow of saliva and helps clean debris from the mouth.

FOODS AS MEDICINE

"Your food shall be your medicine".

— *Hippocrates*

As prosperity increases, the average man and woman are better fed but most of them remain poorly nourished. The progress of civilisation has led to an increasing concentration of population in big cities. As a consequence, man has become divorced from nature and its rich, beautiful bounty, farm fresh foods prepared by nature which meet man's nutritional needs.

Diet plays a decisive role not only in the prevention of diseases but sometimes in curing them also. From ancient times, we in India have endowed food with magical qualities. In Vedic times, food was associated with divine attributes. This tradition was prevalent in other societies as well, in ancient Egypt, for example. Night blindness was a well-recognised disease in ancient Egypt. The cure suggested was to apply to the eyes juice squeezed from cooked liver. The ancient Greeks recommended that the patient should eat cooked liver in addition to applying cooked liver oil or juice to the eyes.

This is a good example of how man discovered the healing powers of food, perhaps initially by accident. Later these patterns became well established and were described in medical texts. The astonishing fact is their proven value in treating disorders primarily caused by lack of food and nutrients.

Another dramatic episode in man's search for a cure is the story of scurvy—a disease characterised by spongy and bleeding gums. It is caused by Vitamin C deficiency. Sailors on long sea voyages, when supplied with canned food, suffered from it. Fresh vegetables, lemons, oranges and other citrus fruits were found to be very effective in preventing and controlling scurvy.

Food has been classified from several points of view: energy giving, body building and protective. Micro and macro nutrients have also been distinguished. Here is one more classification from the angle of using food as medicine. Food may be classified in the categories of fruits, vegetables, cereal grains, pulses, and some other foods. A separate book can be written on the preventive and curative qualities of all the above foods but I shall try to give a brief description of a few items to present a sample of what particular foods can do to keep us healthy. I have tried to include specially those foods which prevent or cure old age diseases like diabetes, heart attack, arthritis etc. or help in delaying the ageing process.

Fruits

Fruits are one of the oldest forms of food known to man. People in ancient times regarded fruits to be endowed with magic or divine properties. They gave them due reverence and dedicated them to gods. Actually fruits are excellent sources of minerals, vitamins and enzymes. They contain fibre and, hence, have laxative effect. They maintain acid-alkaline balance in the body and cater to the body's requirement of natural sugar, vitamins and minerals. As mentioned in the next chapter, fasting is nature's oldest and most effective method of treating diseases and the best way of fasting is fruit juice fasting. Some people past fifty take full meals only once in the day and take fruits in the evening and remain healthy and energetic throughout their lives. Here is a description of some prominent fruits with their curative qualities.

Apple (Seb)

The apple is a native of Eastern Europe and Western Asia but it now grows in abundance in our country as well. It is said that 'an apple a day keeps the doctor away'. It is rich in sugar, calcium, phosphorus, iron, and Vitamin A. It is highly beneficial in the treatment of anaemia. Because of its high content of water and fibre, it treats constipation. It is a natural medicine for stomach disorders.

Apples are of special value to heart patients. They are rich in potassium and phosphorus but low in sodium. Recent research has shown that people who consume plenty of potassium through food items are likely to escape heart attacks. The fruit also plays a useful role in preventing tooth decay. It has a mouth cleansing property that no other fruit possesses. Its acid content preserves teeth and promotes the flow of saliva.

Banana (Kela)

It is one of the oldest and best known fruits of the world. Its original home is believed to be India and Malaysia. It is delicious and seedless and is available in all seasons at a price which is within everybody's reach. It is also very hygienic and germ free as it comes in a germ proof package.

The banana is of great nutritional value. It has a rare combination of energy value tissue-building elements, protein, vitamins and minerals. In combination with milk, it is almost a complete balanced diet. In the traditional medicine system of India and ancient Persia, it was regarded as nature's secret for perpetual youth.

The banana is used as a dietary food against intestinal disorders because of its soft texture and blandness. It is said to contain an unidentified compound called, perhaps jokingly, Vitamin 'U' (against ulcer). It neutralises hyper-acidity and reduces the irritation of ulcer by coating the lining of the stomach.

Bananas are of great value both in constipation and diarrhoea as they normalise colonic functions in the large intestine to absorb large amount of water for proper bowel movements. Their usefulness in constipation is due to their richness in pectin, which is water absorbant and this gives them a bulk producing ability. Mashed banana together with a little salt is a very effective remedy for dysentery.

Grapes (Angoor)

Grapes are one of the most valuable fruits. They are delicious, highly nutritious and most easily digestible. It is a highly valued fruit for its rich content of sugar, which is formed almost entirely by glucose. The glucose is predigested food and is absorbed in the body soon after its consumption. It supplies heat and energy to the body within a short time.

The "grape cure" is perhaps the best of the various fruit cures, proposed from time to time for stomach disorders. Doctors prescribe grape juice five times a day. The treatment lasts for four-to-six weeks. Cellulose, sugar and organic acid in the grapes make it a laxative food. Chronic constipation and dyspepsia are cured by it.

Grapes are highly beneficial in the treatment of heart disease. They tone up the heart and are effective in cardiac pain and palpitation of the heart. They have an exceptional diuretic value on account of the high content of water and potassium salt. Its value in kidney trouble is enhanced by its low albumin and sodium chloride content. Grapes are considered useful in asthma as well. Some physicians are of the opinion that the asthma patient can recover early if kept in a grapes garden.

Indian Gooseberry (Amla)

Amla is a wonderful fruit and one of the precious gifts of nature to man. It is probably the richest known natural source of Vitamin C which is readily assimilated by the human system. It contributes greatly towards health and longevity.

Amla is indigenous to India. It has been used as a valuable ingredient of various medicines from time immemorial. Shustrut, the great Ayurvedic authority, considers it as the best of all acidic fruits and most useful for health and curing disease. Like Ayurvedic physicians, hakims of

Unani medicine also use it very commonly and regard it as a good medicine for heart trouble and other ailments.

Amla is valued chiefly for its high Vitamin C content. This Vitamin C value of Amla increases further when the juice is extracted from the fruit. The best way to take it, with the least loss of Vitamin C, is to eat it raw with a little salt.

Many medicinal values have been attributed to Amla. The fresh fruit is light, laxative and diuretic. It is considered valuable in diabetes. A spoonful of its juice mixed with a cup of fresh bitter gourd (Karela) juice, if taken daily for two months, reduces blood sugar and prevents eye complications in diabetes. It is considered an effective remedy for heart disease as it tones up the functions of all the organs of the body and builds up health. The dried fruit is valuable in diarrhoea and dysentery. Its powder cures chronic constipation. It is an accepted hair tonic and preserves their growth and pigmentation.

Prevents ageing: Amla has revitalising effects. It contains an element which prevents ageing and maintains youthfulness. It improves body resistance and protects against infection. It strengthens the heart, hair and different glands in the body. It is said that the great ancient sage Muni Chayawan rejuvenated himself in his late 70s and regained virility by the use of Amla.

Jambul (Jamun)

The jambul fruit or jamun has been cultivated in the India-Malaysian region for a long time. It grows abundantly during rainy season. The jamun tree is very common and found in most parts of India.

The jamun fruit is regarded in traditional medicine as a curative remedy in diabetes because of its effect on the pancreas. Its seeds contain glucose 'jamboline', which is believed to have the power to check the pathological conversion of starch into sugar in cases of increased

117

production of glucose. They are dried and powdered. This powder in doses of three grams should be given three or four times a day mixed with water. It reduces the quantity of sugar in urine and allays unquenchable thirst.

In Ayurveda, the inner bark of the jamun tree is also used for the treatment of diabetes. The bark is dried and burnt, which produces an ash of white colour. The ash is made into a paste and kept in a bottle. It should be taken in specific quantity in consultation with an Ayurvedic expert.

The jamun fruit is also an effective remedy for bleeding piles. The fruit should be taken with salt every morning for 2 or 3 months in season. It is claimed that its user will be saved from bleeding piles for his entire life.

The jamun fruit should not be consumed in excess. Its excessive use is bad for the throat and chest and may cause cough and accumulation of sputum in lungs.

Mango (Aam)

The mango enjoys a unique status among fruits. It is called the king of fruits. It is indigenous to India and cultivated here for over 4000 years. Besides India, the fruit is widely grown in China, Philippines, Mexico and Brazil. In India alone, there are over 500 varieties of mango.

The mango is used as food in all stages of its development. Green or unripe mango contains a large portion of starch which gradually changes into glucose, sucrose and maltose as the fruit begins to ripen.

The mango is well known for its medicinal properties both in unripe and ripe states. Unripe mango protects men from heatstroke. A drink prepared from unripe mango, mixed with salt and sugar, is an effective remedy against heat and exhaustion. It prevents the loss of salt and iron during summer season due to excessive sweating.

Ripe mangoes are a very effective remedy for night blindness. This disease is caused by the deficiency of Vitamin A and is very common among children. Liberal use of mangoes during the season is very beneficial. The mango-milk treatment is an ideal cure for loss of weight. The mangoes selected should be ripe and sweet. Twice or thrice a day the mango should be taken followed by milk. The mango is rich in sugar but deficient in protein. On the other hand, milk is rich in protein but deficient in sugar. Taken together, they make an ideal diet. If taken for a month, they will improve health, vigour and weight.

Orange (Santra)

The orange is one of the finest gifts of nature. It is the most popular and widespread among the citrus fruits. Though a native of China, now it is widely cultivated .in India. Maharashtra, Sikkim, Assam and Coorg are its cultivation centres.

The orange is rich in protective food ingredients like Vitamins A, B, C and calcium. It also contains sodium, potassium, magnesium, copper, sulphur and chlorine. Its Vitamin C content helps body tissues use the calcium contained in the food.

The orange is a predigested food and the starch of the orange is converted into readily assimilable sugar by the rays of the sun. It is thus readily absorbed in the blood. It produces heat and energy in the body immediately after its use.

Orange is an excellent food in all types of fevers when digestive power of the body is seriously hampered. In chronic dyspepsia, it gives rest to the digestive organs and supplies nutrition in an easily assimilable form.

Orange juice, sweetened with honey, is highly beneficial in heart disease. In cardiac conditions, when only liquid food is permitted, orange juice with honey is a very safe energy-giving food.

Vegetables

Vegetables are important protective food and highly beneficial for the maintenance of health and prevention of diseases.

They contain valuable food ingredients which can be successfully utilised to build up and repair the body.

Food value: Vegetables are valuable in maintaining alkaline reserve in the body. They are valued mainly for their high vitamin and mineral contents. Vitamins A, B and C are contained in vegetables in fair amounts.

It is not the green vegetables only that are useful. Vegetables consisting of starchy roots, such as potatoes, sweet potatoes, the tubers and legumes are also valuable. They are excellent sources of carbohydrates and provide energy to the body.

Natural benefits: To derive maximum benefits of their nutrients, vegetables should be consumed fresh as far as possible. Most vegetables are best consumed in their natural raw state in the form of salads. An important consideration in making salads is that the vegetables should be fresh, crisp and completely dry. If vegetables have to be cooked, it should be ensured that their nutritive value is preserved to the maximum extent possible. The following hints will be useful in achieving this:

1. The vegetables, after a thorough wash, should be cut into as large pieces as possible.

2. The cut pieces should be added to water which has been brought to boiling point and to which salt has been added. This is necessary to avoid loss of B-Complex vitamins and Vitamin C.

3. Only bare minimum water necessary to cover vegetables should be used. Spinach and other tender greens need no water.

4. Vegetables should not be exposed to atmospheric air. They should be covered tightly while cooking.

5. They should be cooked for as short a time as possible. They should be cooked till they are just soft to touch, for easy mastication.

6. They should be served hot.

Bitter Gourd (Karela)

It is a common vegetable cultivated extensively all over India. It also grows in Indonesia, Sri Lanka, Malaysia, Philippines, and China.

The bitter gourd has excellent medicinal properties. It is a laxative, appetising and antipyretic tonic. It is also used in medicines in Asia and Africa.

Curative Properties:

Diabetes: The bitter gourd is specifically used as folk medicine for diabetes. Recent research by a team of British doctors has established that it contains a hypoglycaemic or insulin-like ingredient, designated as plant-insulin, which has been found highly beneficial in lowering the blood and urine sugar levels. It should, therefore, be included liberally in the diet of the diabetic. For better results, the diabetic should take the juice of about four or five fruits every morning on an empty stomach. The seeds of bitter gourd can be added to food in the powdered form. Diabetics can also use bitter gourd in the form of a decoction by boiling the pieces in water or in the form of dry powder.

A majority of diabetics usually suffer from malnutrition as they are usually undernourished. Bitter gourd being rich in all the essential vitamins and minerals, especially Vitamin A, B1, B2, C and iron, its regular use prevents many complications such as hypertension, eye complications, neurotics and defective metabolism of carbohydrates. It increases the body's resistance against infection.

Piles: Juice of the fresh leaves of bitter gourd is valuable in piles. Three teaspoonfuls of leaf juice, mixed with a glassful of butter milk, should be taken every morning for about a month in this condition. A paste of the roots of bitter gourd plant can also be applied over piles with beneficial results.

Bottle Gourd (Ghia or Kaddu)

It is a very common vegetable in India and has been cultivated since time immemorial. It is also cultivated in Asia, Africa and South America.

The cooked vegetable is cooling, diuretic and sedative. It gives a feeling of relaxation after eating. A glassful of fresh juice, mixed with a teaspoonful of lime juice, is useful in urinary disorders. It is a good treatment for burning sensation in the urinary passage due to high acidity of urine. It serves as an alkaline mixture.

Heart disease: Recently it has been claimed that its juice mixed with the juice of ginger (adrak), if taken thrice a day, is a very good medicine for blocked arteries. I have met one or two persons who claimed that after taking the juice for six months or so, their blood cholesterol was reduced and bypass surgery was avoided. The claim is yet to be verified and proved clinically but can be tried under medical supervision. It may contain properties which reduce blood cholesterol and open the clogged blood vessel.

Cabbage (Patta Gobi)

The cabbage is one of the most highly-rated leafy vegetables and a marvellous food item. It is an excellent muscle builder and cleanser. It is chiefly valuable for its high mineral, vitamin and alkaline salts. It can be used raw in the form of salad or can be boiled and cooked. The raw cabbage is more easily digestible than the cooked one.

The cabbage provides roughage and stimulates bowel movement. It is an excellent remedy for constipation. Raw cabbage juice is a miracle cure for duodenal ulcers due to its content of Vitamin U.

Premature ageing: Research has shown that cabbage contains several elements and factors which enhance the immunity of the human body and arrest premature ageing. The vegetable is of great value for persons of advancing age. Some of the elements help prevent the formation of patches on the walls of blood vessels and stones in the gall-bladder. It has been found that a combination of Vitamin B and C in cabbage lends strength to the blood vessels.

Precaution: Cabbage and cabbage juice should never be taken as the main part of diet. Its excessive intake may cause a thyroid disease called goitre.

Carrot (Gajar)

It is a popular vegetable the world over. It is a powerful cleansing food. It is a rich source of Vitamin A. The name carotene, which is a form of pro-vitamin, has been derived from carrot. The carotene is converted into Vitamin A by the liver and it is also stored in our body.

Carrots are rich in sodium, sulphur, chlorine and contain traces of iodine. The mineral contents in carrots lie very close to the skin. Hence they should not be peeled or scrapped off. Carrot juice is known as a 'miracle juice'. It strengthens the eyes and keeps the mucus membranes of all cavities of the body in healthy condition. It is an effective remedy for intestine colic, colitis, appendicitis, peptic ulcer and dyspepsia. Combined with spinach juice and a little lemon juice, it is an effective treatment for constipation.

Fenugreek (Methi)

It is a well-known leafy vegetable and has excellent medicinal properties. It has proteins, calcium, iron and Vitamin C, besides some other nutrients. It is highly beneficial in indigestion, anaemia, stomach disorder and sore throat.

Diabetes: Fenugreek seeds have been found highly effective in the treatment of diabetes. According to a recent report brought out by the Indian Council of Medical Research, fenugreek seeds, when given in varying doses of 25 grams to 100 grams daily, diminish reactive hyperglycaemia in diabetic patients. Levels of glucose, serum cholesterol and triglycerides were also significantly reduced in the diabetic patients when the seeds were consumed, the report said. Quoting researchers at the National Institute of Nutrition, Hyderabad, the report said that the effect of taking fenugreek seeds could be quite dramatic when consumed with 1200-1400 calories diet per day, which is usually recommended for diabetic patients.

Onion (Piyaz)

It is a pungent vegetable of the Lily family. It is considered a food of exceptional value for flavouring and seasoning. The

Sanskrit equivalent for onion is 'palandu' which has been mentioned in the *Garuda Purana*. The great Indian sages, Maharishi Atraya and Lord Dhanwantri, have described the use of onions in detail.

The odour in onion is due to organic sulphur compounds, and is produced only when tissues are cut. Onion contains carbohydrates, Vitamin C and phosphorus, besides iron, calcium, and protein. It is beneficial in respiratory diseases like cough, cold and bronchitis. It is a good cure for cholera, urinary system disorders and skin diseases.

Heart disease: Recent research has established onion as an effective preventive food item against heart attack. Dr. N.N. Gupta of the K.G. Medical College, Lucknow, and a panel of doctors in England, have stated that onion has been found helpful and beneficial in diseases of the heart. According to them, these benefits are due to the presence of essential oil, alipropyl disulphine, catechol, protocatechnic acid, thiopropiono aldehyde, thiocyanate, calcium, iron, phosphorus and vitamins in onion.

Dr. N. Radhakrishnan, Principal of the Trivandrum Medical College and Dr. K. Madhavan Kutty have established, after seven years of research, that to get rid of coronary heart or blood pressure disorders, one should take 100 gms of onion per day. The onion is very valuable in heart diseases as they correct thrombosis and also reduce blood cholesterol.

Bleeding piles: Onion is valuable in bleeding piles. About 30 grams of onions should be finely rubbed in water and 60 grams of sugar added to it. It should be taken twice daily by the patient. It will bring relief within a few days.

Garlic (Lahsun)

It is a vegetable of the onion family. It has been variously described as a food, a herb, a medicinal plant, an antiseptic and a beauty aid as well. It is highly esteemed for its health building qualities. Hippocrates, the father of modern medicine who taught and practised in ancient Athens, recommended the use of this medicine in infectious diseases and intestinal disorders.

Garlic contains iodine, sulphur, phosphorus and Vitamin C, besides carbohydrates and protein. It contains a volatile oil, called allyl sulphade, which is highly antiseptic. It is freely absorbed by the skin and penetrates deeper in tissues. Thus, garlic works as a rejuvenator, removes toxins, stimulates blood circulation and normalises intestinal flora.

High blood pressure: Garlic is regarded as one of the most effective remedies to lower blood pressure. The pressure and tension are reduced because it has the power to ease the spasm of the small arteries. It also slows the pulse and modifies the heart rhythm, besides relieving the symptoms of dizziness, shortness of breath and the formation of gas within the digestive track. Nowadays, garlic capsules are available at chemist shops, the average dosage of two to three capsules a day may be given to cure blood pressure.

Dr. F.G. Piotrowski, working at the University of Geneva, used garlic on 100 patients suffering from abnormally high blood pressure. In about 40 percent of the cases treated, there was a significant reduction in blood pressure within one week of the treatment. Dr. Piotrowski claimed that garlic had a dilatory effect on the blood vessels, that is, it had the effect of making the blood vessels wider, thereby reducing the pressure.

Heart attacks: In a recent study, a West German doctor claimed that garlic may prevent heart attacks. Professor Hans Reuter of Cologne University says that there is proof that garlic helps break up cholesterol in the blood vessels, thus helping in the prevention of hardening of arteries which leads to high blood pressure and heart attacks. If a patient takes garlic after a heart attack, the cholesterol level will come down. The earlier damage may not be repaired but its consumption will minimise the chances of new attacks.

Cancer: Garlic preparations, including extracts and juices, have been used successfully against cancer in both animal and human studies, says Dr. Paavo Airola, a naturopathic physician and nutritionist. A study report tells of mice being infected with cancer cells, some of which were then treated with garlic extract, and some were not. The mice not given garlic died within 16 days, the other mice lived for six months. And recent studies done in Russia have found garlic preparations retarding tumour growth not only in animals, but also in human beings.

Asthma: Three cloves of garlic, boiled in milk, can be used every night with excellent results in asthma. A pod of garlic is peeled and macerated and boiled in 120 ml of pure malt-vinegar. After cooling, it is strained and equal quantity of honey is mixed and preserved in a clean bottle. One or two teaspoons of this syrup taken with fenugreek decoction once in the evening and before retiring, have been found effective in reducing the severity of asthmatic attacks.

Radish (Muli)

It is a commonly used vegetable in India. It is a rich source of iron, calcium and sodium. It also contains Vitamin C and a little Vitamin B. The green leaves of radish are beneficial in jaundice and the seeds of radish are valuable in leucoderma.

Piles: The juice of the fresh root is regarded as an effective food remedy in piles. It should be given in doses of 60 to 90 ml, morning and evening.

Genito-urinary disorders: This juice is also beneficial in the treatment of dysuria or painful urination and strangury or severe urethral pain. It may be given in doses mentioned above and repeated as often as necessary. A cupful of radish leaf juice given once daily for a fortnight acts as a curative medicine in dissolving gravel in urinary tract and inflammation of urinary bladder.

Tomato (Tamatar)

The tomato is one of the most important vegetables in most regions of the world. Only about 130 years back, the tomato was considered poisonous. It was regarded as an acid-forming food. Because of this belief, those suffering from gout, rheumatism, arthritis and general acidosis were advised not to use it. It was also blamed as a cancer culprit. It was also believed that it had no food value and used only to colour and flavour the diet. But the latest studies in nutritional chemistry have established that it has unsurpassable nutritional and health-giving qualities.

Tomato is rich in calcium, phosphorus, Vitamin C and carbohydrate. The carbohydrate in tomato is chiefly in the form of invert sugar, which is the pre-digested form. It is a general stimulant for kidneys and helps to pass away toxins which cause disease. It is essentially an alkaline vegetable. Eating a tomato early in the morning prevents the formation of stone by supplying sufficient quantity of acids, Vitamin A and Vitamin C.

Diabetes: Because of its low carbohydrate contents, it is a very good food for diabetic patients and for those who want to reduce their body weight. It is also very effective in controlling the percentage of sugar in the urine of diabetic patients.

Grain Cereals

Grains are generally classified as the seeds of cereal plants. They are characterised by their smallness, hardness and low water content. Most of them belong to the family of grasses, known scientifically as the family of gramineae.

Food value: The whole grains of all cereals have a similar chemical composition and nutritive value. They are classified as carbohydrate-rich foods, for their average carbohydrate content is 70 percent per 100 gm. They provide energy and also some protein which is usually of good quality. The protein content of grains varies from 11.8 percent for wheat to 8.5 percent for rice per 100 gm. Whole cereals are good sources of calcium and iron but they are totally devoid of ascorbic acid and practically devoid of Vitamin A activity. Yellow maize is the only cereal containing appreciable amounts of carotene. Whole grain cereals also contain significant amounts of B group of vitamins. For a balanced diet, cereals should be supplemented by other proteins, minerals and Vitamin A and C found in nuts, seeds, milk, fruits and fresh green vegetables.

Whole grain cereals play an important role in the diet. If sprouted, they provide an increase in protein balance, as well as in all other nutrients especially Vitamin C. Their complex form of carbohydrate, when in the whole state, is valuable for digestive needs, especially in providing excellent sources of vital fibre.

Rice (Chawal)

Rice is a much revered oriental food and the most important tropical cereal. It is the staple food of about half the human race and is often the main source of calories.

Starch constitutes the bulk of the rice grain. The protein content of rice is lower than that of wheat, but is of superior quality and utilised better by the body than the wheat protein.

The ancient and modern oriental healers through traditional medicines have always advocated the use of natural brown rice as a key to youthful health-building. The processing removes many of the valuable B-Complex vitamins and some of the minerals.

Curative properties: Rice has always been considered a magical healer in the East. It was originally believed to have medicinal values that could restore tranquillity and peace to those who were easily upset. It has been mentioned in early oriental writings that natural whole grain brown rice is a perfect healing food. In the ancient literature of Thailand, Burma, Malaya and Indo-China rice is mentioned as a source of health. It was also revered as a food of divine health and used in religious offerings.

Modern research has confirmed the beliefs of ancient oriental folk physicians that the eating of brown rice is a source of serenity and tranquillity. It has been shown to contain all the elements needed for the maintenance of good health.

Rice is about 98 percent digestible. It is one of the most easily and quickly digested of all foods—being fully digested in an hour. Rice starch is different from other grain starches as it contains 100 percent amylopectin, which is the most completely and rapidly digested grain starch. This makes rice an ideal health food for those who seek speedy and healthy assimilation.

High blood pressure: Rice has a low fat, low cholesterol and low salt content. It makes a perfect diet for those hypertensive persons who have been advised salt-restricted diets. It has been noted by modern researchers that wherever rice is used as the main food, there is a corresponding benefit of youthful vitality and a very low rate of hypertension. Calcium in brown rice, in particular, soothes and relaxes the nervous system and helps relieve the symptoms of high blood pressure.

Kheer—A nutritious diet: The rice diet, in combination with milk, creates a marvellous food. Either fresh milk is taken with each of the rice meals or the rice may be cooked in it. The nutrients in the rice form a unique balance with those in the milk. The two notable amino acids, isoleucine and lysine, in the milk are greatly strengthened by rice protein, thereby enabling them to form stronger body-building blocks. The natural lactic acid in milk works with rice protein to aid in the absorption of iron.

Wheat (Gehun)

Wheat is one of the most common cereals used throughout the world. It is also one of the most valuable cereals and a good source of energy. With its essential coating of bran, vitamins and minerals, it is an excellent health building food.

Food value: Wheat has become the principal cereal, being more widely used for the making of bread than any other cereal because of the quality and quantity of its characteristic protein, called gluten. As it is gluten that makes bread dough stick together and gives it the ability to retain gas, the higher the proportion of gluten in the flour, the better for making leavened bread.

The germ or embryo of the wheat is relatively rich in protein, fat and several of the B vitamins. So is the scutellum in wheat which contains 50 times more thiamin than the whole grain. The outer layers of the endosperm and the aleurone contain a higher concentration of protein, vitamins and phytic acid than the inner endosperm. The inner endosperm contains most of the starch and protein in the grain.

Wheat is usually ground into flour before use as food. In ancient times, wheat grains were crushed between two large stones. This method of stone-grinding preserved all parts of the kernel and the product was called 'whole wheat'. If it is finely ground, it becomes whole wheat flour. The value of stone grinding is that the grain is ground slowly and it remains unheated, and a whole food. In modern times, steel roller mills have superseded stone grinding. These mills grind wheat hundred times faster, but they impoverish the flour by removing the wheat germ, resulting in colossal loss in vitamins and minerals in the refining process.

Curative properties: The wheat, as produced by nature, contains several medicinal properties. Every part of the whole wheat grain supplies elements needed by the human body. Starch and gluten in wheat provide heat and energy, the inner bran coats, phosphates and other mineral salts; the outer bran, the much needed roughage—the indigestible portion which helps easy movement of bowels; the germ, vitamins B and E; and protein of wheat helps build and repair muscular tissue. The wheat germs, which are removed in the process of refining, are also rich in essential Vitamin E, the lack of which can lead to heart disease. The loss of vitamins and minerals in the refined wheat flour has led to widespread prevalence of constipation and other digestive disturbances and nutritional disorders. The whole wheat, which includes bran and wheat germs, therefore, provides protection against diseases such as constipation, inadequate blood flow, heart disease of the colon called diverticulum, appendicitis, obesity and diabetes.

Constipation: The bran of wheat, which is generally discarded in milling of the flour, is more wholesome and nourishing than the flour itself. It is an excellent laxative. The laxative effects of bran are much superior to those of fruits or green vegetables as cellulose of the latter is more easily broken down by bacteria while passing through the intestine. The bran is highly beneficial in the prevention and treatment of constipation due to its concentration of cellulose which forms a bulk mass in the intestines and helps easy evacuation.

Pulses

Pulses may be defined as the dried edible seeds of cultivated legumes. They belong to the family of peas, beans and lentils. The English word 'pulse' is taken from the Latin 'puls', meaning pottage or thick pap. The pulses are a large family and various species are capable of surviving in very different climates and soils.

Pulses are cultivated in all parts of the world, and they occupy an important place in human diet. They, however, make a much more important contribution to the diet of all classes of society in the East than in the West. In India, especially, people who are mostly vegetarian, depend largely on cereals and pulses in their staple food, which serve 'as the main source of dietary protein and energy.

Food value: Pulses contain more protein than any other plant. They serve as a low-cost protein to meet the needs of a large section of the people. They have, therefore, been justifiably described as 'the poor man's meat'. Their low moisture content and hard testa or seed coat permit storage over long periods. In addition to providing dry pulses, many of the crops are grown for their green edible pods and unripe seeds. Nutritionally, immature fruits have distinctly different properties to those of the mature seed. Their protein content is lower but they are relatively richer in vitamins and soluble carbohydrates. The leaves and shoots of some of the crops are used as vegetables.

In general, pulses contain 20 to 28 percent protein per 100 gm. with the exception of soyabean which has as much as 47 percent. Their carbohydrate content is about 60 percent per 100 gm. except soyabean which has about 30 percent. Pulses are also fairly good sources of thiamin and niacin and provide calcium, phosphorus and iron. On an average 100 gm of pulses contain energy 345 kcal, protein 24.5 gm, calcium 140 mg, phosphorus 300 mg, iron 8 mg, thiamin 0.5 mg, riboflavin 0.3 mg and niacin 2 mg.

Curative properties: The nutritive properties of pulses resemble in many respects those of the whole cereal grains; but there are important differences. First, the pulse protein is low in sulphur-containing amino acids, but rich in lysine in which many cereals are deficient. A combination of pulses and cereal proteins may, therefore, have a nutritive value as good as animal proteins. Secondly, pulses as a class are good sources of the B group of vitamins except riboflavin. More important, the greater part of these vitamins present in the harvested seeds is actually consumed. There are no losses comparable with those arising in the milling and cooking of cereals.

Thirdly, although pulses, like cereal grains, are devoid of Vitamin C, large amount of ascorbic acid is formed on germination. Sprouted pulses are, therefore, an important food which will protect against scurvy. Dietitians in Asian and African hospitals make beneficial use of sprouted pulses for their menus, especially when fresh vegetables and fruits are scarce or too expensive.

In healthy condition, the digestion of pulses and the absorption of their principal nutrients is practically complete and nearly as effective as is the assimilation of cereals. Their digestion may, however, be incomplete in gastro-intestinal disorders. Only small quantities of well-cooked pulses should, therefore, be included in the diets of patients with stomach disorders.

Bengal Gram (Chana)

Bengal gram is one of the most important pulses in India. It is consumed in the form of whole dried seeds and in the form of dal, prepared by splitting the seeds in a mill and separating the husk.

Food value: The whole dried Bengal gram seeds are cooked or boiled. They are also consumed raw after soaking them in water. For preparation of dal, the seeds are sprinkled with water and heaped overnight to soften the husk and are then dried before milling. Flour is made by grinding seeds. This flour is one of the main ingredients of many forms of Indian confectionary made with ghee and sugar. It is also used for preparing many tasty snacks like sev, chila and pakoras and curries like koftas. Green pods and tender shoots are used as vegetables.

Curative properties: Bengal gram has many medicinal properties, soaked in water overnight and chewed in the morning with honey, the whole gram seed acts as a general tonic. Sprouted Bengal gram supply plenty of B-Complex and other vitamins. Cooked germinated gram is a wholesome food for children and invalids. However, excessive use of Bengal gram causes indigestion and may precipitate urinary calcium due to high concentration of oxalic acid and form urinary stone of calculi.

Diabetes: Experiments have shown that the intake of water extract of Bengal gram enhances the utilisation of glucose in both the diabetic and the normal person. Tests conducted on chronic diabetic patients, whose insulin requirement was of the order of 40 units a day, when kept on a diet, which included liberal supplements of Bengal gram extract, the condition of the patient improved considerably and his insulin requirement was reduced to about 20 units per day. Diabetic patients who are on a prescribed diet, which does not severely restrict the intake of carbohydrates, but includes liberal amounts of Bengal gram extract, have shown considerable improvement in their fasting blood sugar levels, glucose tolerance, urinary excretion of sugar and general condition.

Anaemia: Fresh juice of Bengal gram leaves is a very rich source of iron. It is, therefore, highly beneficial in the treatment of iron deficiency anaemia. A tablespoonful of fresh juice mixed with honey should be taken in this condition.

Black Gram (Urad)

Black gram is one of the most highly-prized pulses of India. It originated in India where it has been in cultivation from very ancient times. It is cultivated in other Asian countries and in Africa as well but nowhere it is so important as in India.

Curative properties: Black gram is demulcent or soothing and cooling agent. It is an aphrodisiac and nervine tonic. However, excessive use of black gram causes flatulence which can, however, be prevented by adding little hing, pepper and ginger in culinary preparations. It should not be taken by those who are easily predisposed to rheumatic disease and urinary calculi as it contains oxalic acid in high concentration.

Diabetes: Germinated black gram, taken with half a cupful of fresh bitter gourd juice and a teaspoonful of honey, is highly beneficial in the treatment of milder type of diabetes. It should be used once daily for three to four months with restriction of carbohydrates. Even in severe cases, regular use of this combination, with other precautions, is useful as a health-giving food for the prevention of various complications that may arise due to malnutrition in diabetic patients.

Milk

Milk is one of the most common articles of food throughout the world. It occupies a unique position in the maintenance of health and healing disease. It is considered as 'Nature's most nearly perfect food'

The milk of animals has been used by mankind from time immemorial. The milk of cow, buffalow and goat is generally used. In certain places, however, milk of sheep and mare is also used. Cow's milk contains almost twice as much protein as human milk but less sugar. Buffalow's milk contains more fat than cow's milk.

Food value: Milk is regarded as a complete food. It contains protein, fat, carbohydrates, all the known vitamins, various minerals and all the food ingredients considered essential for sustaining life and maintaining health. The protein of milk is of the highest biological value and it contains all the amino acids essential for body building and repair of body cells.

A litre of milk provides all the calcium needed by an individual for one day, practically all the phosphorus, a liberal amount of vitamins A and C, one third or more of the protein, one eighth or more of the iron, at least one fourth of the energy and some of vitamins B, E and D. Milk ranks high in digestibility. Its fat is 99 percent digestible, its protein 97 percent and its carbohydrates 98 percent. Milk is said to require about one and a half hours for digestion. It curdles almost immediately after it reaches the stomach. The organic salts and water begin to be absorbed immediately, while solid matters are passed on to the intestines where the fat is quickly absorbed by the lacteals.

Curative properties: According to Charaka, the great authority on the Indian system of medicine, milk increases strength, improves memory, removes exhaustion, maintains strength and promotes long life. Experiments conducted in modern times have amply corroborated this opinion of Charaka.

Milk is the only article of diet which is well accepted as a wholesome food for persons of all ages, from infancy to old age. It is of special value in feeding infants, toddlers, growing children and expectant and nursing mothers. It is also recommended as a wholesome food for invalids.

Underweight: Milk diet is highly beneficial in the treatment of thinness. If one is considerably below the normal weight, the gain will be from two to four kilograms a week, depending upon the quantity of milk consumed. The body gradually fills out. The eyes become clear and bright and the complexion assumes a healthy colour. The assimilative organs gain renewed energy and power and the gain in the weight is permanent.

Poor blood circulation: An exclusive milk diet is very valuable for those suffering from poor blood circulation. The natural increase in circulation results from the increased amount of fluid assimilated by the stomach and intestines. Hands and feet, which are usually cold in the case of poor circulation, become warm and the patient gets a feeling of well-being within a few days on the milk diet.

Hyperacidity: A milk diet has proved very efficacious in case of hyperacidity and other acid conditions of the stomach. It requires a large amount of acid for its digestion. As milk contains excess of alkaline forming elements, it quickly relieves all acid conditions of the system.

Insomnia: Milk is very valuable in sleeplessness. A glass of milk sweetened with honey, should be taken every night before going to bed in this condition. It acts as a tonic and tranquilliser. Massaging the milk over the soles of the feet has also been found effective.

Respiratory system disorders: Milk has proved useful in respiratory system disorders such as common cold, hoarseness, laryngitis, tonsillitis, bronchitis and asthma. A glassful of pure boiled milk, mixed with a pinch of turmeric powder and few broken pepper, should be taken every night for three nights in these conditions. It will bring beneficial results.

Curd (Dahi)

Curd or yoghurt is a lactic fermentation of milk. It is esteemed for its smoothness and pleasant and refreshing taste. It is a highly health-promoting and therapeutic food.

Food value: Curd is a very nourishing food. It is a valuable source of protein, essential vitamins and minerals. It is also a rich source of calcium and riboflavin. The protein in curd is more readily digested than the protein in milk. It has been estimated that regular milk is only 32 percent digested after an hour in the digestive tract, whereas 91 percent of curd is digested within the same period of time. It is, therefore, an ideal diet for those with sensitive digestive systems, particularly young children and elderly persons.

Curative properties: Although curd has a nutritive content similar to fresh milk, it has extensive special values for therapeutic purposes. During the process of making curd, bacteria convert milk into curd and predigested milk protein. These bacteria then inhibit the growth of hostile or illness-causing bacteria inside the intestinal tract and promote beneficial bacteria needed for digestion. These friendly bacteria facilitate the absorption of minerals, and aid in the synthesis of vitamins of the B group. Buttermilk, which has the same nutritive and curative value as curd, is prepared by churning curd and adding some water and removing the fat in the form of butter.

Gastrointestinal disorders: Apart from the lactic acid organisms placed in milk for the purpose of souring it, the acid of sour milk and its lactose content are important curative factors in a number of diseases. Curd brings relief to patients suffering from gastrointestinal disorders such as chronic constipation and diarrhoea.

Orla Jensen of Copenhagen, author of *Lactic Acid Bacteria*, observes that yoghurt and fermented beverages may be frequently used in case of gastric irritation where other foods cannot be retained by the stomach. The lactic acid, he says, is completely metabolised to carbon dioxide and water is not excreted in the urine. It also does not have any effect on acid base balance in the system. It is, thus, an alkaline food. Besides aiding in the digestion of food, curd decreases dryness and gas in the stomach by helping in secretion of hydrochloric acid, pepsin and renin.

The germs, which give rise to infection and inflammation, such as those which cause appendicitis, diarrhoea and dysentery, cannot thrive in the presence of lactic acid found in curd and buttermilk. Beneficial results have been achieved by the use of buttermilk in cases of colitis. Buttermilk enemas have been found beneficial in the treatment of colitis, chronic constipation, diarrhoea, dysentery, chronic appendicitis and gastric ulcer.

Insomnia: Curd is valuable in the treatment of insomnia. The patient should take plenty of curd and massage it on the head. This will induce sleep.

Premature ageing: Curd has been associated with longevity. Prof. Elic Metchnikoff, a Noble Prize-winning Russian Bacteriologist at the Pasteur Institute, believed that premature old age and decay could be prevented by taking sufficient curd in the daily diet. He made an intensive study of the problem of old age in the early 20th century. He came to the conclusion that the body is slowly being poisoned and its resistance weakened by man's "normal" diet and that this poisoning process could be arrested and the intestinal tract kept healthy by the constant, regular use of yoghurt.

Honey (Shahad)

Honey is one of nature's most splendid gifts to mankind. It possesses unique nutritional and medicinal properties. It is a viscid, saccharine substance, a semi-translucent liquid of a light yellowish-brown colour. It has aromatic odour and sweet acid taste. After some time, it becomes opaque and crystalline. Bees alone are capable of making honey and honeycomb.

The word 'honey' is derived from the Arabic 'han'. This became 'honig' in German and 'hunig' in old English. The word is used in the English language as a term of endearment.

Origin and history: In India, honey has been used for several thousand years as an ingredient for medicines. In Egypt also, it formed the basis of many medical preparations. The ancient Greeks attributed many virtues to it. Hippocrates, the father of modern medicine, prescribed it 2000 years ago to his patients as a remedy for several ailments. He believed that honey, combined with other foods, was nourishing and health giving. Aristotle, the father of natural science, held that its use improved health and prolonged life.

It is well known that the ancient Egyptians and Greeks used honey to embalm their dead. It has a wonderful keeping quality. In a tomb of a queen of Egypt, who was buried over 3,000 years ago, a jar of honey was found which had not undergone any appreciable change in its chemical composition or in its original aroma. It has been recently found that honey retains all its qualities even after 22 years.

Food value: The sugars in honey are glucose, fructose and sucrose. Glucose is the simplest of the sugars. It occurs in the blood of live animals, in fruit and vegetable juice. It restores the oxygen that is replaced by lactic acid when fatigue sets in. Fructose, which is also known as levulose or grape sugar, crystallises more easily than glucose and builds up tissues. Sucrose is a combination of glucose and fructose. Dextrine, which is a gummy substance, is found in small amounts in honey, but it makes honey so digestible.

Latest research indicates that the pollen in honey contains all 22 amino acids, 28 minerals, 11 enzymes, 14 fatty acids and 11 carbohydrates. Unfortunately, much of those nutritive qualities are lost by heating the honey to 150°C for commercial use. Filtering, bottling and cooling to protect its flavours, remove the pollen grains and do not leave the honey as a pure product.

Curative properties: Honey is one of the finest sources of heat and energy. Energy is generated mainly by the carbohydrate foods and honey is one of the most easily digested forms of carbohydrates. It enters directly into the bloodstream because of its dextrine contents and this provides almost instantaneous energy. It is a boon to those with weak digestion. All organs in the body respond favourably when honey is eaten. The famous Roman physician, Galen, has described honey as an all-purpose medicine for all types of diseases. It is now used as a curative and preventive medicine for several ailments.

One spoon of fresh honey, mixed with the juice of half a lemon in a glass of lukewarm water and taken as the first thing in the morning, is an effective remedy for constipation and hyperacidity. Fasting on this honey-lemon juice water is highly beneficial in the treatment of obesity without loss of energy and appetite.

Heart disease: Dr. Arnold Lorand, an eminent nutrition expert, considers honey as the best food for the heart. He observes, "Honey is easily digested and assimilated, it is the best sweet food, as it does not cause flatulence and can prevent it to a certain extent, promoting the activity of the bowels. It can be easily added to the five meals a day. I recommend it in cases of arteriosclerosis and weak hearts. As it would be unwise to leave such a hard working organ as the heart without food over the long hours of the night, I recommend heart patients take, before going to bed, a glass of water with honey and lemon juice in units and also to take it when awaking at night. Honey is useful in cardiac pain and palpitation of the heart."

Anaemia: Honey is remarkable in building haemoglobin in the body. This is largely due to the iron, copper and manganese contained in it. It is beneficial in the treatment of anaemia as it helps maintain the right balance of haemoglobin and red blood corpuscles.

Pulmonary disease: Honey is highly beneficial in the treatment of all diseases of the lungs. It is said if a jug of honey is held under the nose of an asthma patient and he inhales the air that comes into contact with honey, he starts breathing easier and deeper. The effects last for about an hour or so. This is because honey contains a mixture of 'higher' alcohols and ethereal oil and the vapours given off by them are soothing and beneficial for asthma patients. It usually brings relief whether the air flowing over the honey is inhaled or whether it is consumed or taken either in milk or water. Some authorities recommend one-year-old honey for respiratory diseases.

Irritating cough: The use of honey is highly beneficial in the treatment of irritating cough. As a demulcent or soothing agent, it produces a soothing effect on the inflamed mucus membrane of the upper respiratory tract and relieves irritating cough and symptoms like difficulty in swallowing. For the same reason, it is used in the manufacture of various cough mixtures. Honey gargles are also useful in irritant cough.

Insomnia: Honey is beneficial in the treatment of insomnia. It has hypnotic action in bringing sound sleep. It should be taken with water before going to bed in doses of two teaspoonfuls in a big cupful of water. Babies generally fall asleep after taking honey.

Diseases of the stomach: Honey is useful in maintaining the health of the stomach. It tones up the stomach, helps in proper digestion and prevents stomach diseases. It also decreases the overproduction of hydrochloric acid thereby preventing symptoms like nausea, vomiting and heartburn. When putrified faecal matter and undigested foods are present in the alimentary canal, honey acts as a laxative and clears the digestive canal of the waste matter.

Old age: Honey is specially useful in providing energy and heat to the body in old age. It dries up the phlegm and clears the system of mucus to which a person generally falls victim to in old age. One or two teaspoonfuls of honey in a cupful of boiling water, taken while still warm, is a refreshing and strengthening drink.

Dietary Recommendations for Common Health Concerns

■ **Anaemia (Iron deficiency)**

— Eat dry fruits, leafy green vegetables, gur and red meat if you are a non-vegetarian.

— Do some cooking in iron utensils.

— Take Vitamin C (100 mg) with meals.

■ **Arthritis**

— Take banana, cucumber (khira), garlic, tomato, black gram (urad).

■ **Asthma**

— Take beal fruit, grapes, Indian gooseberry (amla), orange, bottle gourd (kaddu), garlic, ginger, mint (pudina), spinach (palak), coconut, honey.

■ **Cancer prevention**

— Avoid saturated vegetable oils and fried foods.

— Reduce animal foods.

— Take plenty of fresh fruits and vegetables.

— Drink green tea regularly.

■ **Cholesterol problems**

— Keep saturated fat intake low: not more than 5 percent of daily caloric intake.

— Increase consumption of fibre.

— Eat garlic and red pepper.

— Eat plenty of fresh fruits and green vegetables.

— Minimum consumption of refined carbohydrates such as maida.

— Eat onion, sunflower seeds, soyabeans, apples.

■ **Constipation**

— Take more fibre, fruits, vegetables, nuts.

— Drink more water.

■ **Chronic fatigue syndrome**

— Decrease protein to 10% of daily caloric intake.

— Eat a variety of fresh fruits and vegetables.

— Eat garlic regularly.

■ **Heart disease**

— Consider a low fat, vegetarian diet as part of a comprehensive heart-healthy lifestyle programme.

— Decrease animal foods and saturated fats.

— Decrease refined carbohydrates.

— Eat plenty of fresh fruits and vegetables.

— Eat whole grains, nuts and seeds.

— Eat garlic regularly.

■ Hypertension

— Increase fruits and vegetables.

— Avoid salt, salted and salty foods.

— Eat garlic regularly, one or two cloves a day.

— Take rice, lemon, apples.

■ Peptic ulcer

— Eat smaller and more frequent meals.

— Avoid tea, coffee etc.

— Avoid alcohol.

— Avoid milk and milk products.

— Eat plenty of fresh fruits and vegetables.

■ Prostate problem

— Decrease intake of animal foods and saturated foods.

— Take plenty of fresh fruits and vegetables including cooked tomatoes.

— Take whole grains, nuts, seeds etc.

— Avoid tea, coffee etc.

FASTING AS A WAY TO PREVENT OLD AGE

"The more you nourish a diseased body, the worse you make it. Food may be your best medicine or medicine will be your food."

— Hippocrates

Ramzan is a month of fasting for the followers of Islam. They take some food before sunrise and for the whole day, don't touch food or water. Despite the fast, they work hard during the whole day and this work sometimes involves hard physical labour. Similarly, among Hindus, Navratras are observed and millions of people abstain from food for nine days taking one meal in the evening. No adverse effect has ever been observed in these people either physically or mentally except perhaps in the case of some very old, sick or weak persons.

The dread of 'growing old' and becoming a burden to oneself and others is one of man's greatest fears. The fear of becoming sick, senile, helpless and unable to care for oneself is rooted deep in every thinking person's mind. Modern man has made many discoveries to rejuvenate himself physically, mentally and spiritually and fasting is being practised from ancient times in almost all religions. But its importance in creating a quality of agelessness, preventing premature ageing and premature death has been recently discovered.

We eat food and as it passes through the body, it must be masticated, digested, assimilated and then the waste is eliminated. We have four organs of elimination: the bowels,

144

kidneys, lungs and the skin. In order for these elimination organs to work perfectly, the body must build a high vital force of body energy reserves.

It takes a tremendous amount of vital force to pass a large meal through the gastrointestinal tract and also eliminate the work via a 30 feet tube that runs from the mouth to the rectum. It also takes a great amount of vital force to pass liquids through 2 million filters of the human kidneys, to make the liver and gall-bladder do their work and also force the lungs to deeply inhale oxygen round the clock.

The instinct that leads us to fast when the body is sick or wounded, resides in the cells of every living being. The reason that sick or wounded animals refuse to eat is that the instinct of self-preservation takes away their hunger and so they will not eat. In this way, the vital force (which would otherwise have to be used in the digestion of food) is concentrated at the site of the injury to remove waste products, thus purifying and healing the body.

Since the infallible intelligence of the living organism withdraws the sensation of hunger when there is an excess of food or when the body has been wounded, the desire to fast begins when either of these happen.

Keep Clean Inside

Ordinarily the basic cause of all diseases is the accumulation of toxic matter in the digestive system. It becomes necessary to regularly cleanse this system. By fasting all body mechanisms which produce blood, flesh, bones or body juice are cleansed and overhauled. During fasts that body energy which was ordinarily employed for nutritional purposes, also becomes available and that too is utilised for elimination of unwholesome and toxic matter. The elderly could change to a diet of fruits and fruit juices only for one or two days. In the alternative, you could take lightly boiled or stewed vegetables only without adding salt. Such a change in diet would do you good and make you feel great.

An Experiment

Dr. S.S.L. Srivastava, M.D., FDMS, FDCN, FASI, Professor and Head of the Department (Medicine), Medical College, Meerut, conducted an experiment in this direction. 75 persons, 59 males and 16 females, their ages ranging from 20 to above 60, kept fast during Navratras, having only water for 8 days. Their pulse rate, blood pressure, weight, hand grip and average sleep hours were examined daily. Their blood sugar, cholesterol, blood urea and lipid profile were also examined in the beginning and at the end of the fast. After the experiment, Dr. Srivastava came to the following conclusions:

1. **Reduction in weight:** It is helpful in various diseases like arthritis, diabetes and cardiovascular diseases. In the older age group, maintenance of optimum body weight prevents traumatic injuries due to fall.

2. **Changes in cholesterol:** There is a favourable change in lipid profile and HDL (good cholesterol) increases while LDL (harmful cholestrol) is reduced.

3. **Immune changes:** There is improvement in immune system which helps in allergic and autoimmune diseases like rheumatoid arthritis, bronchial asthma, eczema, etc.

4. **Role in controlling cancer growth:** During fasting, cancer cells are put to starvation. This causes decrease in cancer cells before they can multiply. Increase in immune system helps in better surveillance of these cells making the body free from abnormal cells before multiplication.

Some other benefits: The memory becomes as sharp as a razor's edge. You can remember names, places and events that go back many years. You have a better capacity for self-education. Education is not a preparation for life, but education is life itself. To grow mentally and spiritually is the greatest goal we humans can have on this earth. So fasting works in three ways: You purify your body physically, mentally and spiritually and, therefore, enjoy super vitality and health. Your mind becomes a sponge which can absorb new facts and knowledge. Greatest of all is the inner peacefulness and spiritual tranquillity that make life worth living. Through fasting, you find peace of mind, the greatest and rarest gift of life.

Eat to live and keep old age away: Food is a blessing to man but becomes a curse if taken in excess. The human body can take a lot of abuse from overfeeding. But there comes a day when the body's digestive system becomes overstuffed, overworked and overwhelmed. It is then that health problems begin.

Digestive troubles plague modern man. Constipation heads the list of his miseries. We often pack our intestines and colon with foods faster than the functions of digestion and elimination can handle. This overstuffing and retention of waste causes putrification and produces gas. This gas pressure causes many miseries in the body. If the gas presses upwards against the diaphragm you may have a simulated heart attack. If it presses against the back muscles, it can cause terrible backaches. It can also cause pounding headache and pains all over the body.

Toxic Acid Crystal Theory and Back Pains

When people take continuous and heavy meals, some toxic residue is left and is concentrated and crystallised as deposits in the moveable joints. It is a very slow process that few sense until the joints start to give trouble. When these calcium-like spurs attach themselves and calcify, then the joints begin to give pains.

The toxic crystals first attack the feet, which have more than 26 moveable bones in each foot. The force of gravity sends the toxic crystals down into the feet. Gradually the feet and ankle start to stiffen, because the toxic acid crystals replace the lubrication in the joints of the feet. They become stiff and tire easily. The toxic acid crystals move upward, causing pain in knees. These move further up and lower back, upper back and even the neck become stiff and give a lot of trouble.

147

Fasting Therapy

Fast has been accepted and recognised as being the oldest form of therapy. Ayurveda prescribes fasting for many diseases. It is mentioned at many places in the Bible. But the fact should be kept in mind that fasting itself is not a cure for any disease or ailment. The purpose of the fast is to allow the body's vital force full range and scope to fulfil its own self-healing, self-repairing and self-rejuvenating functions to the best advantage. Healing is an internal biological function. Fasting gives the body a physiological rest and permits it to be 100% efficient in healing itself.

Subnutrition Diet

Mahatma Gandhi ate a poor man's diet and fasted frequently. He remained healthy and energetic to his last day. The poor in India rarely suffer from hypertension, cardiovascular diseases and diabetes. Dr. Paul C. Bragg, the world famous specialist on Fasting and Life Extension, recounts his unforgettable experience with Gandhiji in the following words:

"The date I met Gandhiji was July 27, 1946, in New Delhi, which would become the capital of the new Republic of India a year and a month later. At Gandhiji's headquarters there, I received permission to accompany this amazing man on a 21-day fasting trip eastward through India's villages, where he would talk with the people and help them with their problems. At that time, the average Indian earned about 10 cents a day and starvation was a way of life. To show he shared their plight, this saintly and compassionate spiritual leader was planning to travel the dusty roads from village to village on foot, without food and only water, for 3 weeks."

"Gandhiji was then 77 years of age and very frail in appearance. But his looks were indeed deceiving. This man was a tower of strength: physically, mentally and spiritually. His stamina, endurance, energy and mental abilities were astounding to everyone."

"The trek began at sun-up. The heat and humidity were the worst I have ever experienced. I have spent time in some of the hottest spots in the world, including Death Valley in California, the Sahara Desert and across North Africa on an 800-mile bicycle trip in intense summer heat. But never once did Gandhiji seem to tire. Never once did he falter in his brisk pace of walking. The only time he sat down was during talks with the villagers. He would speak for 20 minutes, then answer questions for 20 minutes. Then we continued down the hot, dusty road to the next village. Gandhiji ate nothing and drank only water flavoured with lemon and honey."

"Many who tried to travel with him fell by the wayside, suffering from heat and exhaustion. But Gandhiji was inexhaustible. I have been an athlete and hiker all my life, but I have never seen anyone who had the physical stamina and energy as Gandhiji. Each day he walked and talked until sundown before stopping for a rest. During the 21-day fasting walk, I had many talks with Gandhiji on the power of fasting. Of all I learned from him, this statement seems to me the summation:

"All the vitality and energy I have comes to me because my body is purified by fasting."

Walking mile after mile from village to village, he gave the people courage and hope that a better life was coming to them. His internal strength and beautiful pure soul were so powerful that weak people felt strong after seeing him and hearing his words of wisdom. He gave his unlimited strength to the discouraged and the sick. He brought bright light and love where there was darkness."

It is a fact that cutting of calories can increase energy levels, clarity of thinking and perhaps life expectancy as well. But there are a series of caveats:

(*a*) Before you try to make any adjustments in your diet, consult your physician. More harm has been done to people's health by fad diets than perhaps any other single factor.

149

(*b*) Be sure that if you do cut calories you do not cut out those foods that supply you with important vitamins and minerals.

(*c*) Monitor carefully your feelings and energy levels after you reduce your calorie intake. If after a week or so after starting the calorie cut, you feel rundown and fatigued, you may not be consuming enough calories to maintain your necessary energy levels. In such case, feel free to increase your intake of high energy nutritious foods even though this means an increase in your calorie levels.

Fad diet: Taking a particular thing like milk, or fruit only for a long time.

Above all things, you should remember just one thing. You will not help your health or enjoyment of later years by restricting your diet so much that you do not feel up to performing like your old, energetic and active self. As you get older, you should avoid eating too much. But at the same time, it is absolutely essential that you eat enough. Probably the best rule of thumb is **"neither too thin nor too fat"**, **"neither too little nor too much."**

Books on General Health & Yoga

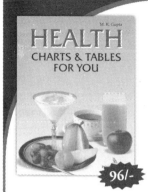

HEALTH
CHARTS & TABLES FOR YOU
M. K. Gupta

96/-

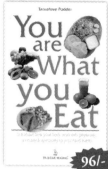

You are What you Eat
Tanushree Podder

96/-

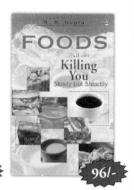

FOODS
that are Killing You
Slowly but Steadily
N. K. Gupta

96/-

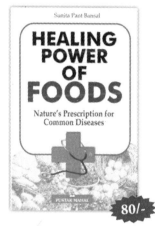

HEALING POWER OF FOODS
Nature's Prescription for Common Diseases
Sunita Pant Bansal

80/-

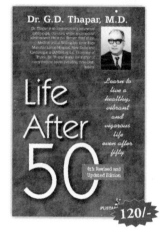

Life After 50
Dr. G.D. Thapar, M.D.

Learn to live a healthy, vibrant and vigorous life even after fifty

4th Revised and Updated Edition

120/-

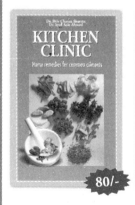

KITCHEN CLINIC
Home remedies for common ailments

80/-

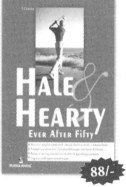

HALE & HEARTY
EVER AFTER FIFTY

88/-

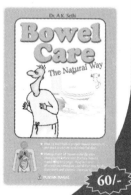

Bowel Care
The Natural Way
Dr. A.K. Sethi

60/-

Postage: Extra